STOP FEMALE FETICIDE

The Preconception and Prenatal Diagnostic Techniques

SAVE THE GIRL CHILD

STOP FEMALE FETICIDE

The Preconception and Prenatal Diagnostic Techniques (Prohibition of Sex Selection) Act, 1994 (Amended Up-to-Date)

Ramesh Verma
MBBS MD (Community Medicine)
Associate Professor
Department of Community Medicine
Pandit Bhagwat Dayal Sharma
Postgraduate Institute of Medical Sciences
Rohtak, Haryana, India

JAYPEE BROTHERS MEDICAL PUBLISHERS (P) LTD
New Delhi • London • Philadelphia • Panama

Jaypee Brothers Medical Publishers (P) Ltd.

Headquarters

Jaypee Brothers Medical Publishers (P) Ltd.
4838/24, Ansari Road, Daryaganj
New Delhi 110 002, India
Phone: +91-11-43574357
Fax: +91-11-43574314
Email: jaypee@jaypeebrothers.com

Overseas Offices

J.P. Medical Ltd.
83, Victoria Street, London
SW1H 0HW (UK)
Phone: +44-2031708910
Fax: +02-03-0086180
Email: info@jpmedpub.com

Jaypee Brothers Medical Publishers Ltd.
The Bourse
111, South Independence Mall East
Suite 835, Philadelphia
PA 19106, USA
Phone: + 267-519-9789
Email: joe.rusko@jaypeebrothers.com

Jaypee Brothers Medical Publishers (P) Ltd.
17/1-B Babar Road, Block-B
Shaymali, Mohammadpur
Dhaka-1207, Bangladesh
Mobile: +08801912003485
Email: jaypeedhaka@gmail.com

Jaypee-Highlights Medical Publishers Inc.
City of Knowledge, Bld. 237, Clayton
Panama City, Panama
Phone: +507-301-0496
Fax: +507-301-0499
Email: cservice@jphmedical.com

Jaypee Brothers Medical Publishers (P) Ltd
Shorakhute
Kathmandu, Nepal
Phone: +00977-9841528578
Email: jaypee.nepal@gmail.com

Website: www.jaypeebrothers.com
Website: www.jaypeedigital.com

Inquiries for bulk sales may be solicited at: jaypee@jaypeebrothers.com

First Edition: **2013**

ISBN 978-93-5090-503-6

Printed at Rajkamal Electric Press, Plot No. 2, Phase-IV, Kundli, Haryana.

Dedicated to

My family

Preface

With the grace of God, the blessing of my parents, good wishes of my wife, brothers, teachers, colleagues and friends, I have been able to write and offer this book before undergraduate, postgraduate medical students and other concerned persons.

The Prenatal Diagnostic Techniques (Regulation and Prevention of Misuse) Act, 1994, was enacted and brought into operation from 1st January, 1996, in order to check female feticide.

The Prenatal Diagnostic Techniques Act and Rules have been amended keeping in view the emerging technologies for selection of sex before and after conception and problems faced in the working of implementation of the Act and certain directions of Hon'ble Supreme Court. These amendments have come into operation with effect from 14th February, 2003.

This book contains full detail of the Preconception and Prenatal Diagnostic Techniques (prohibition of sex selection) Act, 1994 and amended up-to-date. I hope this book will be useful to medical students, radiologists, private practitioners and other concerned persons.

Every attempt has been made to provide full detail, authentic and latest rules and regulations in this book. As with any work, there is always scope of further improvement. For this, I request the readers to send their valuable comments and suggestions.

Ramesh Verma

Acknowledgments

First of all, I would like to thank the Almighty God, who carved out the path for me to tread upon and blessed me with this fortune.

I owe a special debt of gratitude to my teacher Dr Pardeep Khanna, Senior Professor and Head, Department of Community Medicine, Pandit Bhagwat Dayal Sharma Postgraduate Institute of Medical Sciences, Rohtak, Haryana, India, a fount of infinite wisdom, professional competence and constant motivation and inspiration to me.

I sincerely and specially thank Dr Shankar Prinja, Assistant Professor, School of Public Health, Postgraduate Institute of Medical Sciences, Chandigarh, India; Dr Suraj Chawla, Postgraduate Student, Department of Community Medicine, Pandit Bhagwat Dayal Sharma Postgraduate Institute of Medical Sciences, Rohtak, Haryana, India, for constant encouragement, unending moral support and invaluable help.

I registered a deep sense of regards and thankfulness to Dr JS Malik, Senior Professor and Head-II; Professor, Dr BM Vashisht; Professor, Dr MS Punia; Professor, Dr RB Jain; Professor, Dr Neelam Kumar; Professor, Dr Vijay Kumar; Professor, Dr Meena; Dr Meenakshi Kalhan, Associate Professor; and Dr Varun Arora, Assistant Professor; Department of Community Medicine, Pandit Shankar Dayal Sharma Postgraduate Institute of Medical Sciences, Rohtak, Haryana, India, for their support and valuable suggestions.

My sincere thanks to Dr DR Gaur, Professor and Head, Department of Community Medicine, Agroha Medical College, Agroha, Hissar, Haryana, India; Dr NK Saini, Associate Professor, Department of Community Medicine, University College of

Medical Sciences, New Delhi, India; Dr Avneet Singh, Assistant Professor, Department of Community Medicine, Christian Medical College, Ludhiana, Punjab, India; and Dr Manish Goel, Assistant Professor, Department of Community Medicine, Lady Hardinge Medical College, New Delhi, India for their whole-hearted support and encouragement for this difficult task.

I am greatly indebted to my wife Mrs Anita Verma for her unstinting support, painstaking efforts, unending help and encouragement.

Last but not least, I also thank all Senior and Junior Residents, Department of Community Medicine and Mr SK Dua, PA to Director, Pandit Bhagwat Dayal Sharma Post-graduate Institute of Medical Sciences, Rohtak, Haryana, India, for their continuous motivation.

Contents

Introduction

One of the greatest threats to our contemporary civilization is the menace of skewed sex ratio. The increasing imbalance between men and women is leading to many crimes such as illegal trafficking of women, sexual assaults, polygamy and dehumanization of society. These acts have been increasing and making this world unsafe for women. Female feticide is one of the most nefarious crimes on this earth; perhaps what is detestable is that the people who commit crime belong to the educated class. To this menace, our ancestral and biased view about male child, lack of education, ever increasing population and dowry have been good propellants.

A woman when takes birth, she is the daughter, becomes wife after few years and later on she turns into mother of her children. Manu in 200 BC has stated that woman is never independent. As a daughter, she is dependent upon father; as a wife, she is dependent upon husband and in the late years when the king is no more, she is now dependent upon sons.

The issue of female child has always been a question. There is a string preference or "Son syndrome" as male children are considered as assets while female children are considered as liability. Sons are considered essential to keep the family alive; run generation and for that reason all family members pray; "O God, grant the birth of son here and daughter elsewhere."

In India, a girl when getting married is given blessings with hundred sons, never she is blessed with hundred daughters. Birth of a girl in the family is unwelcomed and bringing up of a girl is considered or thought to be "watering in neighbourer garden".

Globally, nature has provided everything in balances whether it's the sex ratio but nature is overruled in India, one of the democratic countries in the world. In the world scenario, India has one of the lowest sex ratio. India is the only country in the world where woman is worshipped as a deity in the past but now in the same country, girl is killed brutally after her birth due to advancement in the technology of medical science like amniocentesis and ultrasonography, she is restricted to give birth. This is fact that her survival is essential for the continuance of human race. To kill girl means to bring an end of the whole of human race.

In India, a Cooperative for Assistance and Relief Everywhere (CARE) project working with adolescent girls noticed about girls that—

"They are often seen only as temporary people, who will cease to be—at least for the father—once they have disappeared in the marriage".

It is a matter of grave concern that today in India, we are discussing on a thing like female feticide. This term is itself envelopes myriads of meanings, it smacks of the fact that:

a. a girl is killed before she is born;
b. that sex of a fetus is determined to identify a female;
c. it acknowledges that there is a technology privy to this heinous crime;
d. there are doctors involved in the first determining the sex of the baby, then carrying out abortion;
e. there is a crime involved in violating not a single but many laws.

Earlier, the most commonly used sex determination test was amniocentesis. It was used as an aid to detect any abnormality in the unborn child. But over the years, it has been used to determine the sex of the fetus. In India, since 1978 the ultrasound technique is being used as a sex determination or sex preselection test. Since then, the test has become extremely popular and has led to a mushrooming of private clinics which perform the test all over the country. Earlier doctors employed the controversial amniocentesis test done between 14 and 18 weeks to determine the sex of the fetus.The ultrasound technique has also been improved. The sex of a fetus can be determined by more sophisticated machines within 13 to 14 weeks of pregnancy by transvaginal sonography and by 14 to 16 weeks through abdominal ultrasound.

The recent technological developments in medical practice combined with a vigorous pursuit of growth of the private health sector have led to the mushrooming of a variety of sex selective services. It has happened not only in urban areas but also deeply rooted within countryside areas.

According to the statistics, nearly 10 million female foetuses have been aborted in the country over the past two decades. Of the 12 million girls born in India, one million do not see their first birthdays. Women are 48.5% of the total population against 51.5% of the men in India (census 2011). During 2001 census, the sex ratio for the total Indian population was 933 (females per thousand males), it increased to the mark of 940 in 2011 census, an increase of seven points. The most disturbing and alarming aspect of census 2011 reports a sharp fall in sex ratio of children (0-6 years age) from 927 in 2001 to 914 in census 2011, a significant decline of 13 points. Although, the overall proportion of children (0-6 years age) has been declining in India, a favorable trend indeed to attribute to the success of family welfare program intervention, however, the declining female child sex ratio over the years, is a disturbing trend.

When the 0 to 6 years ratio is observed statewise during census 2011, it reveals further distressing situation in the states like Punjab (846), Haryana (830), Chandigarh (867), Delhi (866) and Gujarat (886). District wise data on child sex ratio in these States is a quite astounding fact. All these states are prosperous and literacy rate being much higher than rest of the states. This shows that sex ratio has nothing to do with literacy or education. Imbalanced sex ratio at birth, female feticide and higher rate of mortality among girls may perhaps explain this phenomenon.

Facts about Girl Child

- 1 out of every 3 girls does not live to see her 15th birthday
- One-third of these deaths take place at birth
- Every sixth girl child's death is due to gender discrimination
- Females are victimized far more than males during childhood
- 1 out of every 10 women reported some kind of child sexual abuse during childhood, chiefly by known persons
- 1 out of 4 girls is sexually abused before the age of 4
- 19% are abused between the ages of 4 and 8
- 28% are abused between the ages of 8 and 12
- 35% are abused between the ages of 12 and 16
- 1 out of 6 girls will not live to see their 12th birthday
- 3 lakh more girls than boys die every year
- Female mortality exceeds male mortality in 224 out of 402 districts in India
- Death rate among girls below the age of 4 years is higher than that of boys. Even if she escapes infanticide or foeticide, a girl child is less likely to receive immunization, nutrition or medical treatment compared to a male child
- 53% of girls in the age group of 5 to 9 years are illiterate
- Every year 27,06,000 children under 5 years die in India. And the deaths of girl children are higher than those of male children.

'All forms of discrimination against the girl child and violation of her rights shall be eliminated by undertaking strong measures both preventive and punitive within and outside the family. These would relate specifically to strict enforcement of laws against prenatal sex selection and the practices of female foeticide, female infanticide, child marriage, child abuse and child prostitution etc.

The birth of a son is regarded as essential in Hinduism and many prayers and lavish offerings are made in the temples in the hope of having a male child. Modern medical technology is used in the service of this religion driven devaluing of women's and girls. It has been predicted that within next one decade, the ratio would decline to just 500 making this society a criminal society. Either the girls would be purchased from neighboring countries (already happening in Punjab and Haryana) or it would just become a patriarchal society. Women are subjected to cruelty from the male section of this so called advanced society. Even educated women face such treatment, what to talk about uneducated, illiterate women. These days sex determination procedure has proved bane for the girl child. Sex determination tests are forbidden; despite this, they continue to have their hold in this country.

The menace of female feticide started emerging and spreading all over northern and western India and later on all over the country. Today, female feticide is no more an urban phenomenon, rural people are also getting more and more involved in it, and come all the way long to cities to get these tests done.

The state of Punjab in north-west India is known as the "Granary of India" and ranks second only to the National Capital Territory of Delhi in terms of per capita income. Still contrary to popular belief, social development has not kept pace with economic development in Punjab. The discrimination against the girl child is widespread as indicated by the unfavorable sex ratio which is a composite indicator of the status of women. The status of female child index (SFCI, which is a combination of sex ratio of 0 to 9 years age group, school enrolment ratio and child survival ratio) for Punjab, it is 85 to 94.9 on a scale of 100, also mute pointer towards the subjugation of females in this state.

It reflects that the extent of antifemale bias in India is by no means limited to poor income society. Punjab and Haryana, two of the richest states in terms of per capita incomes, have among the lowest female to male sex ratio.

The study carried out in five states - Karnataka, Tamil Nadu, Himachal Pradesh, Uttar Pradesh and Uttaranchal - revealed wide differences in sex ratio in villages of Karnataka and Uttaranchal. The less prosperous villages had a healthy ratio, while their wealthier neighbors, with higher indices of education and development, logged lesser number of girl children. It showed a strong shift from "son preference to active daughter discrimination".

Female infanticide in most places has been replaced by female feticide. Female feticide or sex selective abortion is the elimination of the female fetus in the womb itself. The sex of the fetus is determined by methods like amniocentesis, chorion villus biopsy and now by the most popular technique ultrasonograghy. Once the sex of the fetus is determined, if it is a female fetus, it is aborted. The increase in female feticide has seen the proportionate decrease in female sex ratio. If this decline is not checked, the very delicate equilibrium of nature can be permanently destroyed. In the Indian states of Punjab, Haryana and Uttar Pradesh, mobile vans take sex-detection clinics to outlying villages. "You will find an ultrasound machine even in a village which has a road over which only a bullock cart can go, and electricity to run the machine and nothing else".

Causes of female feticide

1. *Preference of male child:* The traditional preference for sons is deeply rooted in the structure of the society. Since from

earlier times, many rituals were performed when a woman in house was pregnant. It was done in order to pray god for male child. One of the major causes of son preference in India is related to the perceived economic utility of having sons. Compared to daughters, sons provide help in family, farms and businesses, have better earnings prospects in the labor market, and provide support to their parents during old age. Additionally, sons provide the continuation of family names and Hindu custom dictates that only sons can perform the funeral rituals of their parents.

Today, some of the key reasons that exist for the preference of a male child are as follows:

- The tradition of paying dowry at the time of a daughter's marriage is alive and kicking. This amount can be so huge that many parents will go to extreme lengths to avoid having a daughter in the first place.
- A son is seen as someone who can earn and care for his parents in their later years, while a daughter will get married and go away.
- A son can carry on the family name, while a daughter becomes part of her husband's family.
- Girls are seen as consumers, whereas boys are seen as producers.
- Many families consider it a status symbol to have a son, and a point of shame to have a daughter.
- Often, the pressure to bear a male child on the woman is so great that she herself might choose to get sex determination done and abort the baby if it is a girl.
- Illiteracy, poverty and the tag of 'burden' that is assigned to a girl child, makes the desire for a male child even stronger.

2. *Dowry system:* Dowry System is a social evil prevalent in our society since ages. As a result, daughters are considered

to be an economic liability. The dowry system is more rigid in the northern states of India. Many people are not able to get their daughters married because they can't afford dowry. So, they consider it better to kill their baby girl instead of facing all these problems. The evil practice of dowry is widely prevalent in India.

3. *Gender discrimination:* Gender discrimination manifests itself in the form of delay in seeking medical care, seeking care from less qualified doctors and spending lesser money on medicines when a daughter is sick. The extreme disappointment of a mother that girl children adversely affect her ability to breastfeed, which leads to poor nutritional status. That why the prevalence of malnutrition and stunting is higher in girls than boys.
4. *Sexual violence against women:* Sexual offences against women are on rise. Families of victims are not able to maintain their dignity in society.
5. *Women themselves do not want to give birth to a girl child:* This hard fact that women themselves do not want to give birth to a girl child. A survey was conducted at Rajindra hospital, Patiala (Punjab) regarding birth of girl child. It was shocking to know that 56% of girls said that they will not give birth to girl child at any cost and the others were of the view that giving birth to male child will increase their respect in Husband's family.
6. *Advancement of medical technology:* Science is made for the use of man but it is always misused. Amniocentesis technique and ultrasonography were invented to detect any defect in fetus but it is started for determining sex of fetus. Many other techniques are also developed to determine sex of fetus.

Sex ratio is attributable to sex selective abortions (feticides) through sex determination, female infanticide in some states, high mortality in girls during early childhood and sex selective sterilization.

In our country, a girl is worshiped as a *Devi* on one hand and denied her existence on the other hand, as if she has no right to live. Time has perhaps come for us to get rid of male chauvinism, and treat children as gifts of nature regardless of their gender. We cannot imagine a society in the future where there will be only males and no females. The society will be full of crimes and evils. Only legislations enacted on this behalf are not sufficient. Orthodox views regarding women need to be changed. The preconception and prenatal diagnostic techniques (prohibition of sex selection) Act should penalize and punish the violators of this crime strictly. The pernicious acts of female feticide and coercive abortions have to end before women becomes endangered species.

This is an alarming situation that there is an urgent need to turn the minds of people by creating awareness among community that girl child should be accepted as a gift of god. There is need to change in the mind of people that 'Ek Beta Hona Chahiye' and adopt 'Ek Beti Honi Chahiye'. We should not commit same mistakes of our forefathers. Steps should be taken to help the missing girl child for balancing sex-ratio and therefore balancing nature. After all, we are responsible for this imbalance.

Over 250 religious leaders discussed on the ways of ending practice of female feticide. *Akal Takhat* has issued a *Hukamnama* that anyone indulging in unhealthy practice of female feticide would be excommunicated from Sikh religion. The other religious organizations can also play their effective roles besides non-governmental organization (NGOs). The Government has undertaken various measures to address the gender stereotyping and sex roles that have been highlighted in the earlier two reports, through the National Policy on Education, National Policy on Empowerment of Women, which are mainly in the area of educational, creating awareness, gender sensitization, training, mainstreaming gender perspective into main stream in the development process. All forms of media have been utilized to communicate a special message. Customary practices such as dowry, child marriage, sati, sex selective abortion etc. are addressed through legislation and community interactions. These actions and measures are ongoing process which the Government continues to carry on every year to eliminate discriminatory process.

The falling ratio of girl child, crime against women and exploitation of women are blots on civilization and human development. These areas should be high on agenda for policy planners and implementing agencies at all the levels.

Due to excessive female feticide in the northern and western states of India, there were strong agitations and protests to curb the evil of female feticide. The state of Maharashtra became the first in the country to ban prenatal sex determination through the enactment of Maharashtra regulation of prenatal diagnostics techniques Act. Similar efforts at the national level resulted in the enactment of **"The Preconception and Prenatal diagnostic techniques (prohibition of sex selection) Act 1994"**. The act has two aspects viz regulatory and preventive. It seeks to regulate the use of prenatal diagnostic techniques for legal or medical purposes and prevent against misuse for illegal purposes.

THE PRECONCEPTION AND PRENATAL DIAGNOSTIC TECHNIQUES (PROHIBITION OF SEX SELECTION) ACT, 1994

In the recent past, Prenatal diagnostic centers sprang up in the urban areas of the country using prenatal diagnostic techniques for determination of sex of the fetus. Such centers became very popular and their growth was tremendous as the female child is not welcomed with open arms in most of the Indian families. The result was that such centers became centers of females feticide. Such abuse of the technique is against the female sex and affects the dignity and status of women. Various organizations working for the welfare and uplift of the women raised their heads against such an abuse. It was considered necessary to bring out a legislation to regulate the use of, and to provide deterrent punishment to stop the misuse of such techniques. The matter was discussed in Parliament and the Prenatal diagnostic techniques (Regulation and prevention of misuse) bill, 1991 was introduced in the Lok Sabha. The Lok Sabha after discussion adopted a motion for reference of the said bill to a Joint committee of both the Houses of Parliament in September, 1991. The Joint committee presented its report in December, 1992 and on the basis of the recommendations of the committee, the bill was reintroduced in the Parliament.

STATEMENT OF SUBJECTS AND REASONS

It is proposed to prohibit prenatal diagnostic techniques for determination of sex of the fetus leading to female feticide. Such abuse of techniques is discriminatory against the female sex and affects the dignity and status of women. A legislation is required to regulate the use of such techniques and to provide deterrent punishment to stop such inhuman act.

1. The bill, inter alia, provides for:
   - i. Prohibition of the misuse of prenatal diagnostic techniques for determination of sex of fetus, leading to female feticide.
   - ii. Prohibition of advertisement for prenatal diagnostic techniques for detection or determination of sex.
   - iii. Permission and regulation of the use of prenatal diagnostic techniques for the purpose of detection of specific genetic abnormalities or disorders.
   - iv. Permitting the use of such techniques only under certain conditions by the registered institutions.

v. Punishment for violation of the provisions of the proposed legislation.

2. The bill seeks to achieve the above objectives.

ACT 57 OF 1994

The Prenatal diagnostic techniques (Regulation and prevention of misuse) bill having been passed by both the Houses of Parliament received the assent of the President on 20th September, 1994. It came on the statute book as the prenatal diagnostic techniques (Regulations and prevention of misuse) Act, 1994 (57 of 1994). Rules have also been framed under the Act. The Act prohibits determination and disclosure of the sex of fetus. It also prohibits any advertisements related to prenatal determination of sex and prescribes punishment for its contravention. The person who contravenes the provisions of this Act will be punished with imprisonment and fine.

By section 3 of the Prenatal diagnostic techniques (Regulation and prevention of misuse) amendment Act, 2002 (14 of 2003) the nomenclature of the Act has been amended and now it stands as **the preconception and prenatal diagnostic techniques (prohibition of sex selection) Act, 1994 (57 of 1994).**

LIST OF AMENDING ACTS

1. The Prenatal diagnostic techniques (Regulation and prevention of misuse) amendment Act, 2001 (32 of 2001).
2. The Prenatal diagnostic techniques (Regulation and prevention of misuse) amendment Act, 2002 (14 of 2003).
3. The Prenatal diagnostic techniques (Regulation and prevention of misuse) amendment rule, 2003.

chapter

1

Definitions

The preconception and prenatal diagnostic techniques (prohibition of sex selection) Act, 1994

(57 OF 1994) [20th September, 1994]

[An Act to provide for the prohibition of sex selection, before and after conception, and for regulation of prenatal diagnostic techniques for the purposes of detecting genetic abnormalities or metabolic disorders or chromosomal abnormalities or certain congenital malformations or sex linked disorders and for the prevention of their misuse for sex determination leading to female feticide and for matters connected therewith or incidental thereto.]

BE it enacted by Parliament in the Forty-fifth year of the Republic of India as follows:

Preliminary

Short title, extent and commencement

1. This Act may be called [The Preconception and Prenatal Diagnostic Techniques (Prohibition of Sex Selection)] Act, 1994.
2. It shall extend to the whole of India except the State of Jammu and Kashmir.

3. It shall come into force on such date as the Central Government may, by notification in the Official Gazette, appoint.

Definitions

In this Act, unless the context otherwise requires:

a. "**Appropriate Authority**" means the Appropriate Authority appointed under section 17;
b. "**Board**" means the Central Supervisory Board constituted under section 7;
   i. "**conceptus**" means any product of conception at any stage of development from fertilisation until birth including extra embryonic membranes as well as the embryo or fetus;
   ii. "**embryo**" means a developing human organism after fertilization till the end of eight weeks (fifty-six days)
   iii. "**fetus**" means a human organism during the period of its development beginning on the fifty-seventh day following fertilization or creation (excluding any time in which its development has been suspended) and ending at birth;
c. "**Genetic Counseling Center**" means an institute, hospital, nursing home or any place, by whatever name called, which provides for genetic counseling to patients;
d. "**Genetic Clinic**" means a clinic, institute, hospital, nursing home or any place, by whatever name called, which is used for conducting prenatal diagnostic procedures;
   Explanation: For the purpose of this clause, "Genetic Clinic includes a vehicle, where ultrasound machine or imaging machine or scanner or other equipment capable of determining sex of the fetus or a portable equipment which has the potential for detection of sex during pregnancy or selection of sex before and after conception, is used;

e. "**Genetic Laboratory**" means a laboratory and includes a place where facilities are provided for conducting analysis or tests of samples received from Genetic Clinic for prenatal diagnostic test;
f. "**Gynecologist**" means a person who possesses a postgraduate qualification in gynecology and obstetrics;
g. "**Medical geneticist**" includes a person who possesses a degree or diploma certificate in genetics science in the fields of sex selection and prenatal diagnostic techniques or has experience of not less than two years in any of these fields after obtaining:
   i. any one of the medical qualifications recognized under the Indian Medical Council Act, 1956 (102 of 1956); or
   ii. a postgraduate degree in biological sciences;
h. "**Pediatrician**" means a person who possesses a post-graduate qualification in pediatrics;
i. "**Prenatal diagnostic procedures**" means all gynecological or obstetrical or medical procedures such as ultrasonography, fetoscopy, taking or removing samples of amniotic fluid, chorionic villi, embryo blood or any other tissue or fluid of a man, or of a woman before or after conception, for being sent to a Genetic Laboratory or Genetic Clinic for conducting any type of analysis or prenatal diagnostic tests for selection of sex before or after conception.
j. "**Prenatal diagnostic techniques**" includes all prenatal diagnostic procedures and prenatal diagnostic tests;
k. "**Prenatal diagnostic test**" means ultrasonography or any test or analysis of amniotic fluid, chorionic villi, blood or any tissue or fluid of a pregnant woman or conceptus conducted to detect genetic or metabolic disorders or chromosomal abnormalities or congenital anomalies or hemoglobinopathies or sex-linked diseases;

l. "**Prescribed**" means prescribed by rules made under this Act;

m. **"Registered medical practitioner"** means a medical practitioner who possesses any recognized medical qualification as defined in clause (h) of section 2 of the Indian Medical Council Act, 1956, (102 of 1956.) and whose name has been entered in a State Medical Register;

n. "**Regulations**" means regulations framed by the Board under this Act.

o. "**Sex selection**" includes any procedure, technique, test or administration or prescription or provision of anything for the purpose of ensuring or increasing the probability that an embryo will be of a particular sex;

p. "**Sonologist or imaging specialist**" means a person who possesses any one of the medical qualifications recognized under the Indian Medical Council Act, 1956 (102 of 1956) or who possesses a postgraduate qualification in ultrasonography or imaging techniques or radiology;

q. "**State Board**" means a State Supervisory Board or a Union territory Supervisory Board constituted under section 16A;

r. "**State Government**" in relation to Union territory with Legislature means the Administrator of that Union territory appointed by the President under article 239 of Constitution.

Regulation of Genetic Counseling Centers, Genetic Laboratories and Genetic Clinics

chapter 2

On and from the commencement of this Act—

1. No Genetic Counseling Center, Genetic Laboratory or Genetic Clinic unless registered under this Act, shall conduct or associate with, or help in, conducting activities relating to prenatal diagnostic techniques;
2. No Genetic Counseling Center, Genetic Laboratory or Genetic Clinic shall employ or cause to be employed or take services of any person, whether on honorary basis or on payment who does not possess the qualifications as may be prescribed;
3. No medical geneticist, gynecologist, pediatrician, registered medical practitioner or any other person shall conduct or cause to be conducted or aid in conducting by himself or through any other person, any prenatal diagnostic techniques at a place other than a place registered under this Act.

Prohibition of sex selection

No person, including a specialist or a team of specialists in the field of infertility, shall conduct or cause to be conducted or aid in conducting by himself or by any other person, sex selection on a woman or a man or on both or on any tissue, embryo, concepts, fluid or gametes derived from either or both of them.

Prohibition on sale of ultrasound machine, etc. to persons, laboratories, clinics, etc. not registered under the Act

No person shall sell any ultrasound machine or imaging machine or scanner or any other equipment capable of detecting sex of fetus to any Genetic Counseling Center, Genetic Laboratory, Genetic Clinic or any other person not registered under the Act.

chapter 3

Regulation of Prenatal Diagnostic Techniques

On and from the commencement of this Act—

1. No place including a registered Genetic Counseling Center or Genetic Laboratory or Genetic Clinic shall be used or caused to be used by any person for conducting prenatal diagnostic techniques except for the purposes specified in clause (2) and after satisfying any of the conditions specified in clause (3);
2. No prenatal diagnostic techniques shall be conducted except for the purposes of detection of any of the following abnormalities, namely:
   i. chromosomal abnormalities;
   ii. genetic metabolic diseases;
   iii. hemoglobinopathies;
   iv. sex-linked genetic diseases;
   v. congenital anomalies;
   vi. any other abnormalities or diseases as may be specified by the Central Supervisory Board;
3. No prenatal diagnostic techniques shall be used or conducted unless the person qualified to do so, is satisfied for reasons to be recorded in writing that any of the following conditions are fulfilled, namely—
   i. age of the pregnant woman is above thirty-five years;
   ii. the pregnant woman has undergone two or more spontaneous abortions or fetal loss;

iii. the pregnant woman had been exposed to potentially teratogenic agents such as drugs, radiation, infection or chemicals;
iv. the pregnant woman or her spouse has a family history of mental retardation or physical deformities such as, spasticity or any other genetic disease;
v. any other condition as may be specified by the Central Supervisory Board;

Provided that the person conducting ultrasonography on a pregnant woman shall keep complete record thereof in the clinic in such manner, as may be prescribed, and any deficiency or inaccuracy found therein shall amount to contravention of the provision of section 5 or section 6 unless contrary is proved by the person conducting such ultrasonography;

4. No person including a relative or husband of the pregnant woman shall seek or encourage the conduct of any prenatal diagnostic techniques on her except for the purpose specified in clause (2).
5. No person including a relative or husband of a woman shall seek or encourage the conduct of any sex selection technique on her or him or both.

Written consent of pregnant woman and prohibition of communicating the sex of fetus

1. No person referred to in clause (2) of section 3 shall conduct the prenatal diagnostic procedures unless—
   a. he has explained all known side and after effects of such procedures to the pregnant woman concerned;
   b. he has obtained in the prescribed form her written consent to undergo such procedures in the language which she understands;

c. a copy of her written consent obtained under clause (b) is given to the pregnant woman.

2. No person including the person conducting prenatal diagnostic procedures shall communicate to the pregnant woman concerned or her relatives or any other person the sex of the fetus by words, signs or in any other manner.

Determination of sex prohibited

On and from the commencement of this Act—

a. No Genetic Counseling Center or Genetic Laboratory or Genetic Clinic shall conduct or cause to be conducted in its Center, Laboratory or Clinic, prenatal diagnostic techniques including ultrasonography, for the purpose of determining the sex of a fetus;
b. No person shall conduct or cause to be conducted any prenatal diagnostic techniques including ultrasonography for the purpose of determining the sex of a fetus.
c. No person shall, by whatever means, cause or allow to be caused selection of sex before or after conception.

chapter 4

Central Supervisory Board

Constitution of Central Supervisory Board

1. The Central Government shall constitute a Board to be known as the Central Supervisory Board to exercise the powers and perform the functions conferred on the Board under this Act.
2. **The Board shall consist of—**
    a. the Minister in charge of the Ministry or Department of Family Welfare, who shall be the Chairman, ex officio;
    b. the Secretary to the Government of India in charge of the Department of Family Welfare, who shall be the Vice Chairman, ex officio;
    c. three members to be appointed by the Central Government to represent the Ministries of Central Government in charge of Woman and Child Development, Department of Legal Affairs or Legislatives Department in the Ministry of Law and Justice, and Indian System of Medicine and Homeopathy, ex officio;
    d. the Director General of Health Services of the Central Government, ex officio;
    e. ten members to be appointed by the Central Government, two each from amongst—
        i. eminent medical geneticists;

   ii. eminent gynecologists and obstetricians or expert of stri roga or prasuti tantra;
   iii. eminent pediatricians;
   iv. eminent social scientists;
   v. representatives of women welfare organizations;

f. three women Members of Parliament, of whom two shall be elected by the House of the People and one by the Council of States;

g. four members to be appointed by the Central Government by rotation to represent the States and the Union territories, two in the alphabetical order and two in the reverse alphabetical order:

   Provided that no appointment under this clause shall be made except on the recommendation of the State Government or, as the case may be, the Union territory;

h. an officer, not below the rank of a Joint Secretary or equivalent of the Central Government, in charge of Family Welfare, who shall be the Member Secretary, ex officio.

Term of office of members

1. The term of office of a member, other than an ex officio member, shall be—
   a. in case of appointment under clause (e) or clause (f) of subsection (2) of section 7, three years;
      [Provided that the term of office of a member elected under clause (f) of subsection (2) of section 7 shall come to an end as soon as the member become a Minister or Minister of State or Deputy Minister, or the Speaker or the Deputy Speaker of the House of the people, or the Deputy Chairman of the Council of States or ceases to be a member of the House from which he was elected;]

b. in case of appointment under clause (g) of the said subsection, one year.

2. If a casual vacancy occurs in the office of any other members, whether by reason of his death, resignation or inability to discharge his functions owing to illness or other incapacity, such vacancy shall be filled by the Central Government by making a fresh appointment and the member so, appointed shall hold office for the remainder of the term of office of the person in whose place he is so, appointed.
3. The Vice Chairman shall perform such functions as may be assigned to him by the Chairman from time to time.
4. The procedure to be followed by the members in the discharge of their functions shall be such as may be prescribed.

Meetings of the Board

1. The Board shall meet at such time and place, and shall observe such rules of procedure in regard to the transaction of business at its meetings (including the quorum at such meetings) as may be provided by regulations:

   Provided that the Board shall meet at least once in six months.
2. The Chairman, and in his absence the Vice Chairman shall preside at the meetings of the Board.
3. If for any reason the Chairman or the Vice Chairman is unable to attend any meeting of the Board, any other member chosen by the members present at the meeting shall preside at the meeting.
4. All questions which come up before any meeting of the Board shall be decided by a majority of the votes of the members present and voting, and in the event of an equality of votes, the Chairman, or in his absence, the

person presiding, shall have and exercise a second or casting vote.

5. Members other than ex officio members shall receive such allowances, if any, from the Board as may be prescribed.

Vacancies, etc. not to invalidate proceedings of the Board

No act or proceeding of the Board shall be invalid merely by reason of—

a. any vacancy in, or any defect in the constitution of, the Board; or
b. any defect in the appointment of a person acting as a member of the Board; or
c. any irregularity in the procedure of the Board not affecting the merits of the case.

Temporary association of persons with the Board for particular purposes

1. The Board may associate with itself, in such manner and for such purposes as may be determined by regulations, any person whose assistance or advice it may desire in carrying out any of the provisions of this Act.
2. A person associated with it by the Board under subsection (1) for any purpose shall have a right to take part in the discussions relevant to that purpose, but shall not have a right to vote at a meeting of the Board, and shall not be a member for any other purpose.

Appointment of officers and other employees of the Board

1. For the purpose of enabling it efficiently to discharge its functions under this Act, the Board may, subject to such

regulations as may be made in this behalf, appoint (whether on deputation or otherwise) such number of officers and other employees as it may consider necessary:

Provided that the appointment of such category of officers, as may be specified in such regulations, shall be subject to the approval of the Central Government.

2. Every officer or other employee appointed by the Board shall be subject to such conditions of service and shall be entitled to such remuneration as may be specified in the regulations.

Authentication of orders and other instruments of the Board

All orders and decisions of the Board shall be authenticated by the signature of the Chairman or any other member authorised by the Board in this behalf, and all other instruments issued by the Board shall be authenticated by the signature of the Member Secretary or any other officer of the Board authorised in like manner in this behalf.

Disqualifications for appointment as member

A person shall be disqualified for being appointed as a member if, he—

a. has been convicted and sentenced to imprisonment for an offence which, in the opinion of the Central Government, involves moral turpitude; or
b. is an undischarged insolvent; or
c. is of unsound mind and stands so, declared by a competent court; or
d. has been removed or dismissed from the service of the Government or a Corporation owned or controlled by the Government; or

e. has, in the opinion of the Central Government, such financial or other interest in the Board as is likely to affect prejudicially the discharge by him of his functions as a member; or
f. has, in the opinion of the Central Government, been associated with the use or promotion of prenatal diagnostic technique for determination of sex or with any sex selection technique.

Eligibility of member for reappointment

Subject to the other terms and conditions of service as may be prescribed, any person ceasing to be a member shall be eligible for reappointment as such member:

[Provided that no member other than a ex officio members shall be appointed for more than two consecutive terms.]

Functions of the Board

The Board shall have the following functions, namely:

i. to advise the Central Government on policy matters relating to use of prenatal diagnostic techniques, sex selection techniques and against their misuse;
ii. to review and monitor implementation of the Act and the rules made thereunder and recommend to the Central Government changes in the said Act and rules;
iii. to create public awareness against the practice of preconception sex selection and prenatal determination of sex of fetus leading to female feticide;
iv. to lay down code of conduct to be observed by persons working at Genetic Counseling Centers, Genetic Laboratories and Genetic Clinics;
v. to oversee the performance of various bodies constituted under the Act and taken appropriate steps to ensure its proper and effective implementation;
vi. any other functions as may be specified under the Act.

Constitution of State Supervisory Board and Union Territory Supervisory Board

1. Each State and Union territory having Legislature shall constitute a Board to be known as the State Supervisory Board or the Union Territory Supervisory Board, as the case may be, which shall have the following functions:
   i. to create public awareness against the practice of preconception sex selection and prenatal determination of sex of fetus leading to female feticide in the State;
   ii. to review the activities of the Appropriate Authorities functioning in the State and recommend appropriate action against them;
   iii. to monitor the implementation of provisions of the Act and the rules and make suitable recommendations relating thereto, to the Board;
   iv. to send such consolidated reports as may be prescribed in respect of the various activities undertaken in the State under the Act to the Board and the Central Government;
   v. any other functions as may be prescribed under the Act.
2. The State Board shall consists of
   a. the Minister in charge of Health and Family Welfare in the State, who shall be the Chairperson, ex officio;
   b. Secretary in charge of the Department of Health and Family Welfare who shall be the Vice Chairperson, ex officio;
   c. Secretaries or Commissioners in charge of Departments of Women and Child Development, Social Welfare, Law and Indian System of Medicines and Homeopathy, ex officio, or their representatives;

d. Director of Health and Family Welfare or Indian System of medicines and Homeopathy of the State Government, ex officio;
e. three women members of Legislative Assembly or Legislative Council;
f. ten members to be appointed by the State Government out of which two each shall be from the following categories—
   i. eminent social scientists and legal experts;
   ii. eminent women activists from non governmental organizations or otherwise;
   iii. eminent gynecologists and obstetricians or experts of stri roga or prasuti tantra;
   iv. eminent pediatricians or medical geneticists;
   v. eminent radiologists or sonologists;
g. an officer not below the rank of Joint Director in charge of Family Welfare, who shall be the Member Secretary, ex officio.

3. The State Board shall meet at least once in four months.
4. The term of office of a member, other than an ex officio member, shall be three years.
5. If a vacancy occurs in the office of any member other than an ex officio member, it shall be filled by making fresh appointment.
6. If a member of the Legislative Assembly or member of the Legislative Council who is a member of the State Board, becomes Minister or Speaker or Deputy Speaker of the Legislative Assembly or Chairperson or Deputy Chairperson of the Legislative Council, he shall cease to be a member of the State Board.
7. One-third of the total number of members of the State Board shall constitute the quorum.

8. The State Board may coopt a member as and when required, provided that the number of coopted members does not exceed one-third of the total strength of the State Board.
9. The coopted members shall have the same powers and functions as other members, except the right to vote and shall abide by the rules and regulations.
10. In respect of matters not specified in this section, the State Board shall follow procedures and conditions as are applicable to the Board.

Appropriate Authority and Advisory Committee

chapter 5

1. The Central Government shall appoint, by notification in the Official Gazette, one or more Appropriate Authorities for each of the Union territories for the purposes of this Act.
2. The State Government shall appoint, by notification in the Official Gazette, one or more Appropriate Authorities for the whole or part of the State for the purposes of this Act having regard to the intensity of the problem of prenatal sex determination leading to female feticide.
3. The officers appointed as Appropriate Authorities under subsection (1) or subsection (2) shall be,—
    a. when appointed for the whole of the State or the Union territory, consisting of the following three members:
        i. an officer of or above the rank of the Joint Director of Health and Family Welfare Chairperson;
        ii. an eminent women representing women's organization;
        iii. an officer of Law Department of the State or the Union territory concerned:

        Provided that it shall be the duty of the State or the Union territory concerned to constitute multimember State or Union territory level Appropriate Authority within three months of the coming into force of the Prenatal Diagnostic Techniques

(Regulation and Prevention of Misuse) Amendment Act, 2002:

Provided further that any vacancy occurring therein shall be filled within three months of the occurrence.

b. when appointed for any part of the State or the Union territory, of such other rank as the State Government or the Central Government, as the case may be, may deem fit.

4. the Appropriate Authority shall have the following functions, namely:
    a. to grant, suspend or cancel registration of a Genetic Counseling Center, Genetic Laboratory or Genetic Clinic;
    b. to enforce standards prescribed for the Genetic Counseling Center, Genetic Laboratory and Genetic Clinic;
    c. to investigate complaints of breach of the provisions of this Act or the rules made thereunder and take immediate action;
    d. to seek and consider the advice of the Advisory Committee, constituted under subsection (5), on application for registration, and on complaints for suspension or cancellation of registration.
    e. To take appropriate legal action against the use of any sex selection technique by any person at any place, suo motu or brought to its notice and also to initiate independent investigations in such matter;
    f. to create public awareness against the practice of sex selection or prenatal determination of sex;
    g. to supervise the implementation of the provisions of the Act and rules;

h. to recommend to the Board and State Board modifications required in the rules in accordance with changes in technology or social conditions;

i. to take action on the recommendations of the Advisory Committee made after investigation of complaint for suspension or cancellation of registration;

5. The Central Government or the State Government, as the case may be, shall constitute an Advisory Committee for each Appropriate Authority to aid and advise the Appropriate Authority in the discharge of its functions, and shall appoint one of the members of the Advisory Committee to be its Chairman.
6. The Advisory Committee shall consist of—
   a. three medical experts from amongst gynecologists, obstericians, pediatricians and medical geneticists;
   b. one legal expert;
   c. one officer to represent the department dealing with information and publicity of the State Government or the Union territory, as the case may be;
   d. three eminent social workers of whom not less than one shall be from amongst representatives of women's organizations.
7. No person who has been associated with the use or promotion of prenatal diagnostic techniques for determination of sex or sex selection shall be appointed as a member of the Advisory Committee.
8. The Advisory Committee may meet as and when it thinks fit or on the request of the Appropriate Authority for consideration of any application for registration or any complaint for suspension or cancellation of registration and to give advice thereon:

   Provided that the period intervening between any two meetings shall not exceed the prescribed period.

9. The terms and conditions subject to which a person may be appointed to the Advisory Committee and the procedure to be followed by such Committee in the discharge of its functions shall be such as may be prescribed.

Power of Appropriate Authorities

The Appropriate Authorities shall have the powers in respect of the following matters, namely:

a. summoning of any person who is in possession of any information relating to violation of the provisions of the Act or the rules made thereunder;
b. production of any document or material object relating to clause(a);
c. issuing search warrant for any place suspected to be indulging in sex selection techniques or prenatal sex determination;
d. any other matter which may be prescribed.

Registration of Genetic Counseling Centers, Genetic Laboratories and Genetic Clinics

chapter 6

1. No person shall open any Genetic Counseling Center, Genetic Laboratory or Genetic Clinic, including clinic, Laboratory or center having ultrasound or imaging machine or scanner or any other technology capable of undertaking determination of sex of fetus and sex selection or render services to any of them, after the commencement of the Prenatal Diagnostic Techniques (Regulation and Prevention of Misuse) Amendment Act, 2002 unless such Center, Laboratory or Clinic is duly registered under this Act.
2. Every application for registration under subsection (1), shall be made to the Appropriate Authority in such form and in such manner and shall be accompanied by such fees as may be prescribed.
3. Every Genetic Counseling Center, Genetic Laboratory or Genetic Clinic engaged, either partly or exclusively, in counseling or conducting prenatal diagnostic techniques for any of the purposes mentioned in section 4, immediately before the commencement of this Act, shall apply for registration within sixty days from the date of such commencement.
4. Subject to the provisions of section 6, every Genetic Counseling Center, Genetic Laboratory or Genetic Clinic engaged in counseling or conducting prenatal diagnostic techniques shall cease to conduct any such counseling or technique on the expiry of six months from the date of

commencement of this Act unless such Center, Laboratory or Clinic has applied for registration, and is so, registered separately or jointly or till such application is disposed of, whichever is earlier.

5. No Genetic Counseling Center, Genetic Laboratory or Genetic Clinic shall be registered under this Act unless the Appropriate Authority is satisfied that such Center, Laboratory or Clinic is in a position to provide such facilities, maintain such equipment and standards as may be prescribed.

Certificate of registration

1. The Appropriate Authority shall, after holding an inquiry and after satisfying itself that the applicant has complied with all the requirements of this Act and the rules made thereunder and having regard to the advice of the Advisory Committee in this behalf, grant a certificate of registration in the prescribed form jointly or separately to the Genetic Counseling Center, Genetic Laboratory or Genetic Clinic, as the case may be.
2. If, after the inquiry and after giving an opportunity of being heard to the applicant and having regard to the advice of the Advisory Committee, the Appropriate Authority is satisfied that the applicant has not complied with the requirements of this Act or the rules, it shall, for reasons to be recorded in writing, reject the application for registration.
3. Every certificate of registration shall be renewed in such manner and after such period and on payment of such fees as may be prescribed.
4. The certificate of registration shall be displayed by the registered Genetic Counseling Center, Genetic Laboratory

or Genetic Clinic in a conspicuous place at its place of business.

Cancellation or suspension of registration

1. The Appropriate Authority may *suo moto*, or on complaint, issue a notice to the Genetic Counseling Center, Genetic Laboratory or Genetic Clinic to show cause why its registration should not be suspended or cancelled for the reasons mentioned in the notice.
2. If, after giving a reasonable opportunity of being heard to the Genetic Counseling Center, Genetic Laboratory or Genetic Clinic and having regard to the advice of the Advisory Committee, the Appropriate Authority is satisfied that there has been a breach of the provisions of this Act or the rules, it may, without prejudice to any criminal action that it may take against such Center, Laboratory or Clinic, suspend its registration for such period as it may think fit or cancel its registration, as the case may be.
3. Notwithstanding anything contained in subsections (1) and (2), if the Appropriate Authority is of the opinion that it is necessary or expedient so, to do in the public interest, it may, for reasons to be recorded in writing, suspend the registration of any Genetic Counseling Center, Genetic Laboratory or Genetic Clinic without issuing any such notice referred to in subsection (1).

Appeal

The Genetic Counseling Center, Genetic Laboratory or Genetic Clinic may, within thirty days from the date of receipt of the order of suspension or cancellation of registration passed by the Appropriate Authority under section 20, prefer an appeal against such order to—

a. the Central Government, where the appeal is against the order of the Central Appropriate Authority;
b. the State Government, where the appeal is against the order of the State Appropriate Authority, in the prescribed manner.

Offences and Penalties

chapter 7

Prohibition of advertisement relating to preconception and prenatal determination of sex and punishment for contravention

1. No person, organization, Genetic Counseling Center, Genetic Laboratory or Genetic Clinic including Clinic, Laboratory or Center having ultrasound or imaging machine or scanner or any other technology capable of undertaking determination of sex of fetus or sex selection shall issue, publish, distribute, communicate or cause to be issued, published, distributed or communicated any advertisement, in any form, including internet, regarding facilities of prenatal determination of sex or sex selection before conception available at such Center, Laboratory, Clinic or any other place.
2. No person or organization including Genetic Counseling Centre, Genetic Laboratory or Genetic Clinic shall issue, publish, distribute, communicate or cause to be issued, published, distributed or communicated any advertisement in any manner regarding prenatal determination or preconception selection of sex by any means whatsoever, scientific or otherwise.
3. Any person who contravenes the provisions of subsection (1) or subsection (2) shall be punishable with imprisonment

for a term which may extend to three years and with fine which may extend to ten thousand rupees.

Explanation: For the purposes of this section, "advertisement" includes any notice, circular, label, wrapper or any other document including advertisement through internet or any other media in electronic or print form and also includes any visible representation made by means of any hoarding, wall painting, signal, light, sound, smoke or gas.

Offences and penalties

1. Any medical geneticist, gynecologist, registered medical practitioner or any person who owns a Genetic Counseling Center, a Genetic Laboratory or a Genetic Clinic or is employed in such a Center, Laboratory or Clinic and renders his professional or technical services to or at such a Center, Laboratory or Clinic, whether on an honorary basis or otherwise, and who contravenes any of the provisions of this Act or rules made thereunder shall be punishable with imprisonment for a term which may extend to three years and with fine which may extend to ten thousand rupees, and on any subsequent conviction, with imprisonment which may extend to five years and with fine which may extend to fifty thousand rupees.
2. The name of the registered medical practitioner who has been convicted by the court under subsection (1), shall be reported by the Appropriate Authority to the respective State Medical Council for taking necessary action including suspension of the registration if the charges are framed by the court and till the case is dispose of, and on conviction for removal of his name from the register of the Council for a period of five years for the first offence and permanently for the subsequent offence.

3. Any person who seeks the aid of a Genetic Counseling Center, Genetic Laboratory or Genetic Clinic or ultrasound clinic or imaging clinic or of a medical geneticist, gynecologist, sonologist or imaging specialist or registered medical practitioner or any other person for sex selection or for conducting prenatal diagnostic techniques on any pregnant woman for the purposes other than those specified in subsection (2) of section 4, he shall be punishable with imprisonment for a term which may extend to three years and with fine which may extend to fifty thousand rupees for the first offence, and on any subsequent offence with imprisonment which may extend to five years and with fine which may extend to one lakh rupees.
4. For the removal of doubts, it is hereby provided, that the provisions of subsection (3) shall not apply to the woman who was compelled to undergo such diagnostic techniques or such selection.

Presumption in the case of conduct of prenatal diagnostic techniques

Notwithstanding anything contained in the Indian Evidence Act, 1872 (1 of 1872), the court shall presume unless the contrary is proved that the pregnant woman was compelled by her husband or any other relative, as the case may be, to undergo prenatal diagnostic technique for the purposes other than those specified in subsection (2) of section 4 and such person shall be liable for abetment of offence under subsection (3) of section 23 and shall be punishable for the offence specified under that section.

Penalty for contravention of the provisions of the Act or Rules for which no specific punishment is provided

Whoever contravenes any of the provisions of this Act or any rules made thereunder, for which no penalty has been elsewhere provided in this Act, shall be punishable with imprisonment for a term which may extend to three months or with fine, which may extend to one thousand rupees or with both and in the case of continuing contravention with an additional fine which may extend to five hundred rupees for every day during which such contravention continues after conviction for the first such contravention.

Offences by companies

1. Where any offence, punishable under this Act has been committed by a company, every person who, at the time the offence was committed was in charge of, and was responsible to, the company for the conduct of the business of the company, as well as the company, shall be deemed to be guilty of the offence and shall be liable to be proceeded against and punished accordingly:

   Provided that nothing contained in this subsection shall render any such person liable to any punishment, if he proves that the offence was committed without his knowledge or that he had exercised all due diligence to prevent the commission of such offence.
2. Notwithstanding anything contained in subsection (1), where any offence punishable under this Act has been committed by a company and it is proved that the offence has been committed with the consent or connivance of, or is attributable to any neglect on the part of, any director, manager, secretary or other officer of the company, such director, manager, secretary or other officer shall also be

deemed to be guilty of that offence and shall be liable to be proceeded against and punished accordingly.

Explanation: For the purposes of this section,—

a. **"company"** means any body corporate and includes a firm or other association of individuals, and
b. **"director"**, in relation to a firm, means a partner in the firm.

Offence to be cognizable, non-bailable and non-compoundable

Every offence under this Act shall be cognizable, non-bailable and non-compoundable.

Cognizance of offences

1. No court shall take cognizance of an offence under this Act except on a complaint made by—
   a. the Appropriate Authority concerned, or any officer authorised in this behalf by the Central Government or State Government, as the case may be, or the Appropriate Authority; or
   b. a person who has given notice of not less than [fifteen days] in the manner prescribed, to the Appropriate Authority, of the alleged offence and of his intention to make a complaint to the court.
      Explanation—For the purpose of this clause, "person" includes a social organization.
2. No court other than that of a Metropolitan Magistrate or a Judicial Magistrate of the first class shall try any offence punishable under this Act.
3. Where a complaint has been made under clause (b) of subsection (1), the court may, on demand by such person, direct the Appropriate Authority to make available copies of the relevant records in its possession to such person.

chapter 8

Miscellaneous

Maintenance of records

1. All records, charts, forms, reports, consent letters and all other documents required to be maintained under this Act and the rules shall be preserved for a period of two years or for such period as may be prescribed:

   Provided that, if any criminal or other proceedings are instituted against any Genetic Counseling Center, Genetic Laboratory or Genetic Clinic, the records and all other documents of such Center, Laboratory or Clinic shall be preserved till the final disposal of such proceedings.
2. All such records shall, at all reasonable times, be made available for inspection to the Appropriate Authority or to any other person authorized by the Appropriate Authority in this behalf.

Power to search and seize records, etc.

1. If the Appropriate Authority has reason to believe that an offence under this Act has been or is being committed at any Genetic Counseling Center, Genetic Laboratory or Genetic Clinic, or any other place, such Authority or any officer authorized in this behalf may, subject to such rules as may be prescribed, enter and search at all reasonable times with such assistance, if any, as such Authority or

officer considers necessary, such Genetic Counseling Center, Genetic Laboratory or Genetic Clinic or any other place and examine any record, register, document, book, pamphlet, advertisement or any other material object found therein and seize and seal the same if such Authority or officer has reason to believe that it may furnish evidence of the commission of an offence punishable under this Act.

2. The provisions of the Code of Criminal Procedure, 1973 (2 of 1974) relating to searches and seizures shall, so, far as may be, apply to every search or seizure made under this Act.

Protection of action taken in good faith

No suit, prosecution or other legal proceeding shall lie against the Central or the State Government or the Appropriate Authority or any officer authorized by the Central or State Government or by the Authority for anything which is in good faith done or intended to be done in pursuance of the provisions of this Act.

Removal of difficulties

1. If any difficulty arises in giving effect to the provisions of the Prenatal Diagnostic Techniques (Regulation and Prevention of Misuse) Amendment Act, 2002, the Central Government may, by order published in the Official Gazette, make such provisions not inconsistent with the provisions of the said Act as appear to be necessary or expedient for removing the difficulty:

   Provided that no order shall be made under this section after the expiry of the period of three years from the date of commencement of the Prenatal Diagnostic Techniques

(Regulation and Prevention of Misuse) Amendment Act, 2002.

2. Every order made under this section shall be laid, as soon as may be after it is made, before each House of Parliament.

Power to make rules

1. The Central Government may make rules for carrying out the provisions of this Act.
2. In particular and without prejudice to the generality of the foregoing power, such rules may provide for—
    i. the minimum qualifications for persons employed at a registered Genetic Counseling Center, Genetic Laboratory or Genetic Clinic under clause (2) of section 3;
        - the manner in which the person conducting ultrasonography on a pregnant woman shall keep record thereof in the clinic under the proviso to subsection (3) of section 4
    ii. the form in which consent of a pregnant woman has to be obtained under section 5;
    iii. the procedure to be followed by the members of the Central Supervisory Board in the discharge of their functions under subsection (4) of section 8;
    iv. allowances for members other than ex officio members admissible under sub section (5) of section 9;
        a. code of conduct to be observed by persons working at Genetic Counseling Centers, Genetic Laboratories and Genetic Clinics to be laid down by the Central Supervisory Board under clause (iv) of section 16;
        b. the manner in which reposts shall be furnished by the State and Union Territory Supervisory Boards

to the Board and the Central Government in respect of various activities undertaken in the State under the Act under clause(iv) of subsection (1) of section 16A;

c. empowering the Appropriate Authority in any other matter under clause (d) of section 17A;

v. the period intervening between any two meetings of the Advisory Committee under the proviso to sub section (8) of section 17;

vi. the terms and conditions subject to which a person may be appointed to the Advisory Committee and the procedure to be followed by such Committee under subsection (9) of section 17;

vii. the form and manner in which an application shall be made for registration and the fee payable thereof under subsection (2) of section 18;

viii. the facilities to be provided, equipment and other standards to be maintained by the Genetic Counseling Center, Genetic Laboratory or Genetic Clinic under subsection (5) of section 18;

ix. they form in which a certificate of registration shall be issued under subsection (1) of section 19;

x. the manner in which and the period after which a certificate of registration shall be renewed and the fee payable for such renewal under subsection (3) of section 19;

xi. the manner in which an appeal may be preferred under section 21;

xii. the period up to which records, charts, etc. shall be preserved under subsection (1) of section 29;

xiii. the manner in which the seizure of documents, records, objects, etc. shall be made and the manner in which seizure list shall be prepared and delivered to the person from whose custody such documents, records or objects were seized under subsection (1) of section 30;

xiv. any other matter that is required to be, or may be, prescribed.

Power to make regulations

The Board may, with the previous sanction of the Central Government, by notification in the Official Gazette, make regulations not inconsistent with the provisions of this Act and the rules made thereunder to provide for—

a. the time and place of the meetings of the Board and the procedure to be followed for the transaction of business at such meetings and the number of members which shall form the quorum under sub-section (1) of section 9;
b. the manner in which a person may be temporarily associated with the Board under sub section (1) of section 11;
c. the method of appointment, the conditions of service and the scales of pay and allowances of the officer and other employees of the Board appointed under section 12;
d. generally for the efficient conduct of the affairs of the Board.

Rules and regulations to be laid before Parliament

Every rule and every regulation made under this Act shall be laid, as soon as may be after it is made, before each House of Parliament, while it is in session, for a total period of thirty days which may be comprised in one session or in two or more successive sessions, and if, before the expiry of the session immediately following the session or the successive sessions aforesaid, both Houses agree in making any modification in the rule or regulation or both Houses agree that the rule or regulation should not be made, the rule or regulation shall thereafter have effect only in such modified form or be of no effect, as the case may be; so, however, that any such modification or annulment shall be without prejudice to the validity of anything previously done under that rule or regulation.

The Preconception and Prenatal Diagnostic Techniques (Prohibition of Sex Selection) Rules, 1996

chapter 9

Short title and commencement

1. These rules may be called the preconception and prenatal diagnostic techniques (prohibition of sex selection) Rules, 1996.
2. They shall come into force on the date of their publication in the Official Gazette.

Definitions

In these rules, unless the context otherwise requires:

a. **"Act"** means The Prenatal Diagnostic Techniques (Regulation and Prevention of Misuse) Act, 1994 (57 of 1994);
b. **"Employee"** means a person working in or employed by a Genetic Counseling Center, a Genetic Laboratory or a Genetic Clinic, or an Ultrasound Clinic and Imaging Center and includes those working on part-time, contractual, consultancy, honorary or on any other basis;
c. **"Form"** means a form appended to these rules;
d. **"Schedule"** means a Schedule appended to these rules;
e. **"Section"** means a section of the Act;
f. Words and expressions used herein and not defined in these rules but defined in the Act, shall have the meanings, respectively, assigned to them in the Act.

Minimum requirements

1. The minimum qualifications of the employees, the minimum equipment and minimum place for a Genetic Counseling Center, Genetic Laboratory and Genetic Clinic shall be as specified in Schedules I, II and III.
2. Where an institute, hospital, nursing home, or any place, by whatever name called, provides services jointly of Genetic Counseling Center, Genetic Laboratory and Genetic Clinic, or any combination of these, it shall conform to the requirements as specified in Schedules I, II and III.

Sale of ultrasound machines/ imaging machines

1. No organization including a commercial organization or a person, including manufacturer, importer, dealer or supplier of ultrasound machines/imaging machines or any other equipment, capable of detecting sex of fetus, shall sell, distribute, supply, rent, allow or authorize the use of any such machine or equipment in any manner, whether on payment or otherwise, to any Genetic Couseling Center, Genetic Laboratory, Genetic Clinic, Ultrasound Clinic, Imaging Center or any other body or person unless such Center, Laboratory, Clinic, body or person is registered under the Act.
2. The provider of such machine/equipment to any person/ body registered under the Act shall send to the concerned State/UT Appropriate Authority and to the Central Government, once in three months a list of those to whom the machine/equipment has been provided.
3. Any organization or person, including manufacturer, importer, dealer or supplier of ultrasound machine/ imaging machines or any other equipment capable of

detecting sex of fetus selling, distributing, supplying or authorizing, in any manner, the use of any such machine or equipment to any Genetic Counseling Center, Genetic Laboratory, Genetic Clinic, Ultrasound Clinic, Imaging Center or any other body or person registered under the Act shall take an affidavit from the Genetic counseling Center, Genetic Laboratory, Genetic Clinic, Ultrasound Clinic, Imaging Center or any other body or person purchasing or getting authorization for using such machine/equipment that the machine/equipment shall not be used for detection of sex of fetus or selection of sex before or after conception.

Registration of genetic counseling center, genetic laboratory, genetic clinic, ultrasound clinic and imaging center

1. An application for registration shall be made to the Appropriate Authority, in duplicate, in Form A, duly accompanied by an affidavit containing—
   i. an undertaking to the effect that the Genetic Center/Laboratory/Clinic/Ultrasound Clinic/Imaging Center/Combination thereof, as the case may be, shall not conduct any test or procedure, by whatever named called, for selection of sex before or after conception or for detection of sex of fetus except for diseases specified in section 4 (2) nor shall the sex of fetus be disclosed to any body;
   ii. an undertaking to the effect that the Genetic Center/Laboratory/Clinic/Ultrasound Clinic/Imaging Center/Combination thereof, as the case may be, shall display prominently a notice that they do not conduct any technique, test or procedure, etc. by whatever name

called, for detection of sex of fetus or for selection of sex before or after conception

2. The Appropriate Authority, or any person in his office authorized in this behalf, shall acknowledge receipt of the application for registration, in the acknowledgement slip provided at the bottom of Form A, immediately if delivered at the office of the Appropriate Authority, or not later than the next working day if received by post.

Application fee

1. Every application for registration under rule 4 shall be accompanied by an application fee of:
   a. Rs. 3000.00 for Genetic Counseling Center; Genetic Laboratory; Genetic Clinic, Ultrasound Clinic or Imaging Center.
   b. Rs. 4000.00 for an institute, hospital, nursing home, or any place providing jointly the service of a Genetic Counseling Center, Genetic Laboratory and Genetic Clinic, Ultrasound Clinic or Imaging Center or any combination thereof.

      Provided that if an application for registration of any Genetic Clinic/Laboratory/Center, etc. has been rejected by the Appropriate Authority, no fee shall required to be paid on re-submission of the application by the applicant for the same body within 90 days of rejection. Provided further that any subsequent application shall be accompanied with the prescribed fee. Application fee once paid will not be refunded.
2. The application fee shall be paid by a demand draft drawn in favor of the Appropriate Authority, on any scheduled bank payable at the headquarters of the Appropriate Authority concerned. The fees collected by the Appropriate

Authorities for registration of Genetic Counseling Center, Genetic Laboratory, Genetic Clinic, Ultrasound Clinic and Imagining Center or any other body or person under sub-rule (1), shall be deposited by the Appropriate Authority concerned in a bank account opened in the name of the official designation of the Appropriate Authority concerned and shall be utilized by the Appropriate Authority in connection with the activities connected with implementation of the provisions of the Act and these rules.

Certificate of registration

1. The Appropriate Authority shall, after making such enquiry and after satisfying itself that the applicant has complied with all the requirements, place the application before the Advisory Committee for its advice.
2. Having regard to the advice of the Advisory Committee the Appropriate Authority shall grant a certificate of registration, in duplicate, in Form B to the applicant. One copy of the certificate of registration shall be displayed by the registered [Genetic Counseling Center, Genetic Laboratory or Genetic Clinic, Ultrasound Clinic or Imaging Center] at a conspicuous place at its place of business:

   Provided that the Appropriate Authority may grant a certificate of registration to a Genetic Laboratory or a Genetic Clinic to conduct one or more specified prenatal diagnostic tests or procedures, depending on the availability of place, equipment and qualified employees, and standards maintained by such laboratory or clinic.
3. If, after enquiry and after giving an opportunity of being heard to the applicant and having regard to the advice of the Advisory Committee, the Appropriate Authority is

satisfied that the applicant has not complied with the requirements of the Act and these rules, it shall, for the reasons to be recorded in writing, reject the application for registration and communicate such rejection to the applicant as specified in Form C.

4. An enquiry under subrule (1), including inspection at the premises of the Genetic Counseling Center, Genetic Laboratory or Genetic Clinic, Ultrasound Clinic or Imaging Center shall, be carried out only after due notice is given to the applicant by the Appropriate Authority.
5. Grant of certificate of registration or rejection of application for registration shall be communicated to the applicant as specified in Form B or Form C, as the case may be, within a period or ninety days from the date of receipt of application for registration.
6. The certificate of registration shall be nontransferable. In the event of change of ownership or change of management or on ceasing to function as a Genetic Counseling Center, Genetic Laboratory or Genetic Clinic, Ultrasound Clinic or Imaging Center, both copies of the certificate of registration shall be surrendered to the Appropriate Authority.
7. In the event of change of ownership or change of management of the Genetic Counseling Center, Genetic Laboratory or Genetic Clinic, Ultrasound Clinic or Imaging Center, the new owner or manager of such Center, Laboratory or Clinic shall apply afresh for grant of certificate of registration.

Validity of registration

Every certificate of registration shall be valid for a period of five years from the date of its issue.

Renewal of registration

1. An application for renewal of certificate of registration shall be made in duplicate in Form A, to the Appropriate Authority thirty days before the date of expiry of the certificate of registration. Acknowledgement of receipt of such application shall be issued by the Appropriate Authority in the manner specified in subrule (2) of rule 4.
2. The Appropriate Authority shall, after holding an enquiry and after satisfying itself that the applicant has complied with all the requirements of the Act and these rules, and having regard to the advice of the Advisory Committee in this behalf, renew the certificate of registration, as specified in Form B, for a further period of five years from the date of expiry of the certificate of registration earlier granted.
3. If, after enquiry and after giving an opportunity of being heard to the applicant and having regard to the advice of the Advisory Committee, the Appropriate Authority is satisfied that the applicant has not complied with the requirements of the Act and these rules, it shall, for reasons to be recorded in writing, reject the application for renewal of certificate of registration and communicate such rejection to the applicant as specified in Form C.
4. The fees payable for renewal of certificate of registration shall be one half of the fees provided in subrule (1) of rule 5.
5. On receipt of the renewed certificate of registration in duplicate or on receipt of communication of rejection of application for renewal, both copies of the earlier certificate of registration shall be surrendered immediately to the Appropriate Authority by the Genetic Counseling Center, Genetic Laboratory or Genetic Clinic, Ultrasound Clinic or Imaging Center.

6. In the event of failure of the Appropriate Authority to renew the certificate of registration or to communicate rejection of application for renewal of registration within a period of ninety days from the date of receipt of application for renewal of registration, the certificate of registration shall be deemed to have been renewed.

Maintenance and preservation of records

1. Every Genetic Counseling Center, Genetic Laboratory and Genetic Clinic, Ultrasound Clinic and Imaging Center shall maintain a register showing, in serial order, the names and addresses of the men or women given genetic counseling, subjected to prenatal diagnostic procedures or prenatal diagnostic tests, the names of their spouse or fathers, and the date on which they first reported for such counseling, procedure or test.
2. The record to be maintained by every Genetic Counseling Center, in respect of each woman counseled shall be as specified in Form D.
3. The record to be maintained by every Genetic Laboratory, in respect of each man or woman subjected to any prenatal diagnostic procedure/technique/test, shall be as specified in Form E.
4. The record to be maintained by every Genetic Clinic, in respect of each man or woman subjected to any prenatal diagnostic procedure/technique/test, shall be as specified in Form F.
5. The Appropriate Authority shall maintain a permanent record of applications for grant or renewal of certificate of registration as specified in Form H. Letters of intimation of every change of employee, place, address, and equipment installed shall also be preserved as permanent records.

6. All case related records, forms of consent, laboratory results, microscopic pictures, sonographic plates or slides, recommendations and letters shall be preserved by the Genetic Counseling Center, Genetic Laboratory, Genetic Clinic, Ultrasound Clinic or Imaging Center for a period of two years from the date of completion of counseling, prenatal diagnostic procedure or prenatal diagnostic test, as the case may be. In the event of any legal proceedings, the records shall be preserved till the final disposal of legal proceedings, or till the expiry of the said period of two years, whichever is later.
7. In case the Genetic Counseling Center or Genetic Laboratory or Genetic Clinic, Ultrasound Clinic or Imaging Center maintains records on computer or other electronic equipment, a printed copy of the record shall be taken, and preserved after authentication by a person responsible for such record.
8. Every Genetic Counseling Center, Genetic Laboratory, Genetic Clinic, Ultrasound Clinic and Imaging Center shall send a complete report in respect of all preconception or pregnancy related procedures/techniques/tests conducted by them in respect of each month by 5th day of the following month to the concerned Appropriate Authority.

Conditions for conducting prenatal diagnostic procedures

1. Before conducting preimplantation genetic diagnosis, or any prenatal diagnostic technique/test/procedure such as aminocentesis, chorionic villi biopsy, fetoscopy, fetal skin or organ biopsy or cordocentsis, a written consent, as specified in Form G, in a language the person undergoing such procedure understands, shall be taken from her/him.

Provided that where a Genetic Clinic has taken a sample of any body tissue or body fluid and sent it to a Genetic Laboratory for analysis or test, it shall not be necessary for the Genetic Laboratory to obtain a fresh consent in Form G.

Any person conducting ultrasonography/image scanning on a pregnant woman shall give a declaration on each report on ultrasonography/image scanning that he/she has neither detected nor disclosed the sex of fetus of the pregnant woman to any body. The pregnant woman shall before undergoing ultrasonography/image scanning declare that she does not want to know the sex of her fetus.

2. All the State Governments and Union Territories may issue translation of Form G in languages used in the State or Union Territory and where no official translation in a language understood by the pregnant woman is available, the Genetic Clinic may translate Form G into a language she understands.

Facilities for inspection

1. Every Genetic Counseling Center, Genetic Laboratory, Genetic Clinic, Ultrasound Clinic, Imaging Center, Nursing Home, Hospital, Institute or any other place where any of the machines or equipments capable of performing any procedure, technique or test capable of prenatal determination of sex or selection of sex before or after conception is used, shall afford all reasonable facilities for inspection of the place, equipment and records to the Appropriate Authority or to any other person authorized by the Appropriate Authority in this behalf for registration of such institutions, by whatever name called, under the Act, or for detection of misuse of such facilities or advertisement therefore or for selection of sex before or after conception or for

detection/disclosure of sex of fetus or for detection of cases of violation of the provisions of the Act in any other manner.

2. The Appropriate Authority or the officer authorized by it may seal and seize any ultrasound machine, scanner or any other equipment, capable of detecting sex of fetus, used by any organization, if the organization has not got itself registered under the Act. These machines of the organizations may be released, if such organization pays penalty equal to five times of the registration fee to the Appropriate Authority concerned and give an undertaking that it shall not undertake detection of sex of fetus or selection of sex before or after conception.

Procedure for search and seizure

1. The Appropriate Authority or any officer authorized in this behalf may enter and search at all reasonable times any Genetic Counseling Center, Genetic Laboratory, Genetic Clinic, Ultrasound Clinic, Imaging Center or Ultrasound Clinic in the presence of two or more independent witness for the purposes of search and examination of any record, register, document, book, pamphlet, advertisement, or any other material object found therein and seal and seize the same, if there is reason to believe that it may furnished evidence of commission of an offence punishable under the Act.

   Explanation: In these rules

   1. 'Genetic Laboratory/Genetic Clinic/Genetic Counseling Center' would include an Ultrasound Center/ Imaging Center/nursing home/hospital/institute or any other place, by whatever name called, where any of the machines or equipments capable of selection of sex before or after conception or performing any procedure technique or test for prenatal detection of sex of fetus, is used;

   2. 'Material object' would include records, machines and equipment;
   3. 'Seize' and 'seizure' would include 'seal' and 'sealing' respectively;

2. A list of any document, record, register, book, pamphlet, advertisement or any other material object found in the Genetic Counseling Center, Genetic Laboratory, Genetic Clinic, Ultrasound Clinic or Imaging Center and seized shall be prepared in duplicate at the place of effecting the seizure. Both copies of such list shall be signed on every page by the Appropriate Authority or the officer authorized in this behalf and by the witnesses to the seizure:

   Provided that the list may be prepared, in the presence of the witnesses, at a place other than the place of seizure if, for reasons to be recorded in writing, it is not practicable to make the list at the place of effecting the seizure.

3. One copy of the list referred to in subrule (2) shall be handed over, under acknowledgement, to the person from whose custody the document, record, register, book, pamphlet, advertisement or any other material object have been seized:

   Provided that a copy of the list of such document, record, register, book, pamphlet, advertisement or other material object seized may be delivered under acknowledgement, or sent by registered post to the owner or manager of the Genetic Counseling Center, Genetic Laboratory, Genetic Clinic, Ultrasound Clinic or Imaging Center, if no person acknowledging custody of the document, record, register, book, pamphlet, advertisement or other material object seized is available at the place of effecting the seizure.

4. If any material object seized is perishable in nature, the Appropriate Authority, or the officer authorized in this behalf shall make arrangements promptly for sealing,

identification and preservation of the material object and also convey it to a facility for analysis or test, if analysis or test be required:

Provided that the refrigerator or other equipment used by the Genetic Counseling Center, Genetic Laboratory, Genetic Clinic, Ultrasound Clinic or Imaging Center for preserving such perishable material object may be sealed until such time as arrangements can be made for safe removal of such perishable material object and in such eventuality, mention of keeping the material object seized, on the premises of the Genetic Counseling Center, Genetic Laboratory or Genetic Clinic shall be made in the list of seizure.

5. In the case of noncompletion of search and seizure operation, the Appropriate Authority or the officer authorized in this behalf may make arrangements, by way of mounting a guard or sealing of the premises of the Genetic Counseling Center, Genetic Laboratory, Genetic Clinic, Ultrasound Clinic or Imaging Center, for safe keeping, listing and removal of documents, records, book or any other material object to be seized, and to prevent any tampering with such documents, records, books or any other material object.

Intimation of changes in employees, place or equipment

Every Genetic Counseling Center, Genetic Laboratory, Genetic Clinic, Ultrasound Clinic or Imaging Center shall intimate every change of employee, place, address, and equipment installed, to the Appropriate Authority within a period of thirty days of such change.

Conditions for analysis or test and prenatal diagnostic procedures

1. No Genetic Laboratory shall accept for analysis or test any sample, unless referred to it by a Genetic Clinic.
2. Every prenatal diagnostic procedure shall invariably be immediately preceded by locating the fetus and placenta through ultrasonography, and the prenatal diagnostic procedure shall be done under direct ultrasonographic monitoring so, as to prevent any damage to the fetus and placenta.

Meetings of the Advisory Committees

The intervening period between any two meetings of Advisory Committees constituted under subsection (5) of Section 17 to advise the Appropriate Authority shall not exceed sixty days.

Allowances to members of the Central Supervisory Board

1. The ex officio members, and other Central and State Government officers appointed to the Board will be entitled to Travelling Allowance and Daily Allowance for attending the meetings of the Board as per the Travelling Allowance rules applicable to them.
2. The nonofficial members appointed to, and Members of Parliament elected to, the Board will be entitled to Travelling Allowance and Daily Allowance for attending the meetings of the Board as admissible to nonofficial and Members of Parliament as the case may be, under the Travelling Allowances rules of the Central Government.

Public information

1. Every Genetic Counseling Center, Genetic Laboratory, Genetic Clinic, Ultrasound Clinic or Imaging Center shall prominently display on its premises a notice in English, and in the local language or languages for the information of the public, to effect that disclosure of the sex of the fetus is prohibited under law.
2. At least one copy each of the Act and these rules shall be available on the premises of every Genetic Counseling Center, Genetic Laboratory, Genetic Clinic, Ultrasound Clinic or Imaging Center and shall be made available to the clientele on demand for perusal.
3. The Appropriate Authority, the Central Government, the State Government, and the Government/Administration of the Union Territory may publish periodically lists of registered Genetic Counseling Centers, Genetic Laboratories, Genetic Clinics, Ultrasound Clinic or Imaging Center and findings from the reports and other information in their possession, for the information of the public and for use by the experts in the field.

Code of conduct to be observed by persons working at genetic counseling centers, genetic laboratories, genetic clinics, ultrasound clinics, imaging centers, etc.

All persons including the owners, employee or any other persons associated with Genetic Counseling Centers, Genetic Laboratories, Genetic Clinic, Ultrasound Clinics, Imaging Centers registered under the Act/these rules shall:

i. not conduct or associate with, or help in carrying out detection or disclosure of sex of fetus in any manner;
ii. not employ or cause to be employed any person not possessing qualifications necessary for carrying out prenatal diagnostic techniques/procedures, techniques and tests including ultrasonography;
iii. not conduct or cause to be conducted or aid in conducting by himself or through any other person any techniques or procedure for selection of sex before or after conception or for detection of sex of fetus except for the purposes specified in subsection (2) of section 4 of the Act;
iv. not conduct or cause to be conducted or aid in conducting by himself or through any other person any techniques or test or procedure under the Act at a place other than a place registered under the Act/these rules;
v. ensure that no provision of the Act and these rules are violated in any manner;
vi. ensure that the person, conducting any techniques, test or procedure leading to detection of sex of fetus for purposes not covered under section 4 (2) of the Act or selection of sex before or after conception, is informed that such procedures lead to violation of the Act and these rules which are punishable offences;
vii. help the law enforcing agencies in bring to book the violators of the provisions of the Act and these rules;
viii. display his/her name and designation prominently on the dress worn by him/her;
ix. write his/her name and designation in full under his/her signature;
x. on no account conduct or allow/cause to be conducted female feticide;
xi. not commit any other act of professional misconduct.

Appeals

1. Anybody aggrieved by the decision of the Appropriate Authority at subdistrict level may appeal to the Appropriate Authority at district level within 30 days of the order of the subdistrict level Appropriate Authority.
2. Anybody aggrieved by the decision of the Appropriate Authority at district level may appeal to the Appropriate Authority at State/UT level within 30 days of the order of the district level Appropriate Authority.
3. Each appeal shall be disposed of by the District Appropriate Authority or by the State/Union Territory Appropriate Authority, as the case may be, within 60 days of its receipt.
4. If an appeal is not made within the time as prescribed under subrule (1), (2) or (3), the Appropriate Authority under that subrule may condone the delay in case he/she is satisfied that appellant was prevented for sufficient cause from making such appeal.

chapter 10

The Prenatal Diagnostic Techniques (Regulation and Prevention of Misuse) Amendment Act, 2002

(14 of 2003) [17th January, 2003]

An Act further to amend the Prenatal Diagnostic Techniques (Regulation and Prevention of Misuse) Act, 1994.

BE it enacted by Parliament in the Fifty-third year of the Republic of India as follows:

Short title and commencement

1. This Act may be called the Prenatal Diagnostic Techniques (Regulation and Prevention of Misuse) Amendment Act, 2002.
2. It shall come into force on such date as the Central Government may, by notification in the Official Gazette, appoint.

Substitution of long title

In the Prenatal Diagnostic Techniques (Regulation and Prevention of Misuse) Act, 1994 (57 of 1994) (hereinafter referred to as the principal Act), for the long title, the following long title shall be substituted, namely:

"An Act to provide for the prohibition of sex selection, before or after conception, and for regulation of prenatal diagnostic techniques for the purposes of detecting genetic abnormalities or metabolic disorders or chromosomal abnormalities or certain congenital malformations or sex linked disorders and for the prevention of their misuse for sex determination leading to female feticide and for matters connected therewith or incidental thereto".

Amendment of section 1

In section 1 of the principal Act, in subsection *(1)*, for the words and brackets "the Prenatal Diagnostic Techniques (Regulation and Prevention of Misuse)," the words and brackets "the Preconception and Prenatal Diagnostic Techniques (Prohibition of Sex Selection)" shall be substituted.

Amendment of section 2

In section 2 of the principal Act,

i. after clause (b), the following clauses shall be inserted, namely—

   '(ba) *conceptus* means any product of conception at any stage of development from fertilization until birth including extra embryonic membranes as well as the embryo or fetus;

   (bb) *embryo* means a developing human organism after fertilisation till the end of eight weeks (fifty-six days);

   (bc) *fetus* means a human organism during the period of its development beginning on the fifty-seventh day following fertilization or creation (excluding any time in which its development has been suspended) and ending at the birth;

ii. in clause (d), the following *Explanation* shall be added, namely:
'*Explanation*: For the purpose of this clause, "Genetic Clinic" includes a vehicle, where ultrasound machine or imaging machine or scanner or other equipment capable of determining sex of the fetus or a portable equipment which has the potential for detection of sex during pregnancy or selection of sex before conception, is used;'

iii. in clause (e), the following *Explanation* shall be added, namely:
'*Explanation:* For the purposes of this clause "Genetic Laboratory" includes a place where ultrasound machine or imaging machine or scanner or other equipment capable of determining sex of the fetus or a portable equipment which has the potential for detection of sex during pregnancy or selection of sex before conception, is used;'

iv. for clause(g), the following clause shall be substituted, namely:
(g) *medical geneticist* includes a person who possesses a degree or diploma in genetic science in the fields of sex selection and prenatal diagnostic techniques or has experience of not less than two years in any of these fields after obtaining
   a. any one of the medical qualifications recognized under the Indian Medical Council Act, 1956 (102 of 1956); or
   b. a postgraduate degree in biological sciences;

v. for clause *(i)*, the following clause shall be substituted, namely:
(i) prenatal diagnostic procedures means all gynecolo-gical or obstetrical or medical procedures such as ultrasonography, fetoscopy, taking or removing samples of amniotic fluid, chorionic villi, embryo, blood or any

other tissue or fluid of a man, or of a woman before or after conception, for being sent to a Genetic Laboratory or Genetic Clinic for conducting any type of analysis or prenatal diagnostic tests for selection of sex before or after conception;'

vi. for clause (*k*), the following clause shall be substituted, namely:

(*k*) *prenatal diagnostic test* means ultrasonography or any test or analysis of amniotic fluid, chorionic villi, blood or any tissue or fluid of a pregnant woman or conceptus conducted to detect genetic or metabolic disorders or chromosomal abnormalities or congenital anomalies or hemoglobinopathies or sex linked diseases;'

vii. after clause (n), the following clauses shall be inserted, namely:

(o) *sex selection* includes any procedure, technique, test or administration or prescription or provision of anything for the purpose of ensuring or increasing the probability that an embryo will be of a particular sex;

(p) "sonologist or imaging specialist" means a person who possesses any one of the medical qualifications recognised under the Indian Medical Council Act, 1956 (102 of 1956) or who possesses a postgraduate qualification in ultrasonography or imaging techniques or radiology;

(q) *State Board* means a State Supervisory Board or a Union territory Supervisory Board constituted under section 16 A;

(r) *State Government* in relation to Union territory with Legislature means the Administrator of that Union territory appointed by the President under article 239 of the Constitution'.

Amendment of section 3

In section 3 of the principal Act, for clause (2), the following clause shall be substituted, namely:

"*(2)* no Genetic Counseling Center or Genetic Laboratory or Genetic Clinic shall employ or cause to be employed or take services of any person, whether on honorary basis or on payment who does not possess the qualifications as may be prescribed".

Insertion of new sections 3A and 3B

After section 3 of the principal Act, the following sections shall be inserted, namely:

"3A. Prohibition of sex selection: –No person, including a specialist or a team of specialists in the field of infertility, shall conduct or cause to be conducted or aid in conducting by himself or by any other person, sex selection on a woman or a man or on both or on any tissue, embryo, conceptus, fluid or gametes derived from either or both of them.

3B. Prohibition on sale of ultrasound machine, etc. to persons, laboratories, clinics, etc. not registered under the Act. –No person shall sell any ultrasound machine or imaging machine or scanner or any other equipment capable of detecting sex of fetus to any Genetic Counseling Center, Genetic Laboratory, Genetic Clinic or any other person not registered under the Act".

Amendment of section 4

In section 4 of the principal Act, for clauses (3) and (4), the following clauses shall be substituted, namely:

"(3) no prenatal diagnostic techniques shall be used or conducted unless the person qualified to do so, is satisfied for reasons to be recorded in writing that any of the following conditions are fulfilled namely:

i. age of the pregnant woman is above thirty-five years,
ii. the pregnant woman has undergone two or more spontaneous abortions or fetal loss;
iii. the pregnant woman had been exposed to potentially teratogenic agents such as, drugs, radiation, infection or chemicals;
iv. the pregnant woman or her spouse has a family history of mental retardation or physical deformities such as, spasticity or any other genetic disease;
v. any other condition as may be specified by the Board: Provided that the person conducting ultrasonography on a pregnant woman shall keep complete record thereof in the clinic in such manner, as may be prescribed, and any deficiency or inaccuracy found therein shall amount to contravention of the provisions of section 5 or section 6 unless contrary is proved by the person conducting such ultrasonography;

(4) no person including a relative or husband of the pregnant woman shall seek or encourage the conduct of any prenatal diagnostic techniques on her except for the purposes specified in clause (2);

(5) no person including a relative or husband of a woman shall seek or encourage the conduct of any sex selection technique on her or him or both".

Amendment of section 5

In section 5 of the principal Act, for subsection (2), the following subsection shall be substituted, namely:

"(2) No person, including the person conducting prenatal diagnostic procedures shall communicate to the pregnant woman concerned or her relatives or any other person the sex of the fetus by words, signs, or in any other manner".

Amendment of section 6

In section 6 of the principal Act, after clause (b), the following clause shall be inserted, namely:

"(c) no person shall, by whatever means, cause or allow to be caused selection of sex before or after conception."

Amendment of section 7

In section 7 of the principal Act

i. in subsection (2), for clause (*c*), the following clause shall be substituted, namely—
   "(*c*) three members to be appointed by the Central Government to represent the Ministries of Central Government in charge of Women and Child Development, Department of Legal Affairs or Legislative Department in the Ministry of Law and Justice, and Indian System of Medicine and Homeopathy, ex officio";
ii. in clause (*e*), for sub clause (*ii*), the following sub clause shall be substituted, namely:
   "(*ii*) eminent gynaecologist and obstetrician or expert of stri roga or prasuti tantra".

Amendment of section 14

In section 14 of the principal Act, for clause (*f*), the following clause shall be substituted, namely—

"(f) has, in the opinion of the Central Government, been associated with the use or promotion of prenatal diagnostic technique for determination of sex or with any sex selection technique".

Amendment of section 15

In section 15 of the principal Act, the following proviso shall be inserted, namely:

"Provided that no member other than an ex officio member shall be appointed for more than two consecutive terms".

Substitution of new section for section 16

For section 16 of the principal Act, the following section shall be substituted, namely:

"16. Functions of the Board—The Board shall have the following functions, namely:

i. to advise the Central Government on policy matters relating to use of prenatal diagnostic techniques, sex selection techniques and against their misuse;
ii. to review and monitor implementation of the Act and rules made thereunder and recommend to the Central Government changes in the said Act and rules.
iii. to create public awareness against the practice of pre-conception sex selection and prenatal determination of sex of fetus leading to female feticide;
iv. to lay down code of conduct to be observed by persons working at Genetic Counseling Centers, Genetic Laboratories and Genetic Clinics;
v. to oversee the performance of various bodies constituted under the Act and take appropriate steps to ensure its proper and effective implementation;
vi. any other functions as may be prescribed under the Act".

Insertion of new section 16A

After section 16 of the principal Act, the following section shall be inserted, namely:

"16A, Constitution of State Supervisory Board and Union territory Supervisory Board.

1. Each State and Union territory having Legislature shall constitute a Board to be known as the State Supervisory Board or the Union territory Supervisory Board, as the case may be, which shall have the following functions:
   i. to create public awareness against the practice of preconception sex selection and prenatal determination of sex of fetus leading to female feticide in the State;
   ii. to review the activities of the Appropriate Authorities functioning in the State and recommend appropriate action against them;
   iii. to monitor the implementation of provisions of the Act and the rules and make suitable recommendations relating thereto, to the Board;
   iv. to send such consolidated reports as may be prescribed in respect of the various activities undertaken in the State under the Act to the Board and the Central Government;
   v. any other functions as may be prescribed under the Act.
2. The State Board shall consist of:
   a. the Minister in charge of Health and Family Welfare in the State, who shall be the Chairperson, ex officio;
   b. Secretary in charge of the Department of Health and Family Welfare who shall be the Vice Chairperson, ex officio;
   c. Secretaries or Commissioners in charge of Departments of Women and Child Development, Social Welfare, Law and Indian System of Medicines and Homeopathy, ex officio, or their representatives;
   d. Director of Health and Family Welfare or Indian System of Medicines and Homeopathy of the State Government, ex officio;

e. three women members of Legislative Assembly or Legislative Council;
f. ten members to be appointed by the State Government out of which two each shall be from the following categories:
   i. eminent social scientists and legal experts;
   ii. eminent women activists from nongovernmental organizations or otherwise;
   iii. eminent gynaecologists and obstetricians or experts of stri roga or prasuti tantra;
   iv. eminent pediatricians or medical geneticists;
   v. eminent radiologists or sonologists;
g. an officer not below the rank of Joint Director incharge of Family Welfare, who shall be the Member Secretary, ex officio

3. The State Board shall meet at least once in four months.
4. The term of office of a member, other than an ex officio member, shall be three years.
5. If a vacancy occurs in the office of any member other than an ex officio member, it shall be filled by making fresh appointment.
6. If a member of the Legislative Assembly or member of the Legislative Council who is a member of the State Board, becomes Minister or Speaker or Deputy Speaker of the Legislative Assembly or Chairperson or Deputy Chairperson of the Legislative Council, she shall cease to be a member of the State Board.
7. One-third of the total number of members of the State Board shall constitute the quorum.
8. The State Board may coopt a member as and when required, provided that the number of coopted members does not exceed one-third of the total strength of the State Board.
9. The coopted members shall have the same powers and functions as other members, except the right to vote and shall abide by the rules and regulations.

10. In respect of matters not specified in this section, the State Board shall follow procedures and conditions as are applicable to the Board".

Amendment of section 17

In section 17 of the principal Act,

i. in subsection (*3*), for clause (*a*), the following clause shall be substituted, namely:
"(*a*) when appointed for the whole of the State or the Union territory, consisting of the following three members:
   i. an officer of or above the rank of the Joint Director of Health and Family Welfare Chairperson;
   ii. an eminent woman representing women's organization;
   iii. an officer of Law Department of the State or the Union territory concerned:

   Provided that it shall be the duty of the State or the Union territory concerned to constitute multi member State or Union territory level Appropriate Authority within three months of the coming into force of the Prenatal Diagnostic Techniques (Regulation and Prevention of Misuse) Amendment Act, 2002:

   Provided further that any vacancy occurring therein shall be filled within three months of the occurrence";
ii. in subsection (*4*), after clause (*d*), the following clauses shall be inserted, namely:
"(e) to take appropriate legal action against the use of any sex selection technique by any person at any place, suo motu or brought to its notice and also to initiate independent investigations in such matter;
(*f*) to create public awareness against the practice of sex selection or prenatal determination of sex;

(g) to supervise the implementation of the provisions of the Act and rules;

(*h*) to recommend to the Board and State Boards modifications required in the rules in accordance with changes in technology or social conditions;

(*i*) to take action on the recommendations of the Advisory Committee made after investigation of complaint for suspension or cancellation of registration";

iii. for subsection (*7*), the following sub section shall be substituted, namely:

"(*7*) No person who has been associated with the use or promotion of prenatal diagnostic techniques for determination of sex or sex selection shall be appointed as a member of the Advisory Committee".

Insertion of new section 17A

After section 17 of the principal Act, the following section shall be inserted, namely:

"17A. Powers of Appropriate Authorities—The Appropriate Authority shall have the powers in respect of the following matters, namely:

a. summoning of any person who is in possession of any information relating to violation of the provisions of this Act or the rules made thereunder;
b. production of any document or material object relating to clause (a);
c. issuing search warrant for any place suspected to be indulging in sex selection techniques or prenatal sex determination;
d. any other matter which may be prescribed".

Amendment of section 18

In section 18 of the principal Act, for subsection (*1*), the following subsection shall be substituted, namely:

"(1) No person shall open any Genetic Counseling Center, Genetic Laboratory or Genetic Clinic, including clinic, laboratory or center having ultrasound or imaging machine or scanner or any other technology capable of undertaking determination of sex of fetus and sex selection, or render services to any of them, after the commencement of the Prenatal Diagnostic Techniques (Regulation and Prevention of Misuse) Amendment Act, 2002 unless such center, laboratory or clinic is duly registered under the Act".

Substitution of new section for section 22

For section 22 of the principal Act, the following section shall be substituted, namely:

"22. Prohibition of advertisement relating to preconception and prenatal determination of sex and punishment for contravention.

1. No person, organization, Genetic Counseling Center, Genetic Laboratory or Genetic Clinic, including clinic, laboratory or center having ultrasound machine or imaging machine or scanner or any other technology capable of undertaking determination of sex of the fetus or sex selection shall issue, publish, distribute, communicate or cause to be issued, published, distributed or communicated any advertisement, in any form, including internet, regarding facilities of prenatal determination of sex or sex selection before conception available at such center, laboratory, clinic or at any other place.
   "Advertisement" includes any notice, circular, label wrapper or other document and also includes any visible representation made by means of any light, sound, smoke or gas.
2. No person or organization including Genetic Counseling Center, Genetic Laboratory or Genetic Clinic shall issue,

publish, distribute, communicate or cause to be issued, published, distributed or communicated any advertisement in any manner regarding prenatal determination or preconception selection of sex by any means whatsoever, scientific or otherwise.

3. Any person who contravenes the provisions of subsection (1) or subsection (2) shall be punishable with imprisonment for a term which may extend to three years and with fine which may extend to ten thousand rupees.

   Explanation: For the purposes of this section, 'advertisement' includes any notice, circular, label, wrapper or any other document including advertisement through internet or any other media in electronic or print form and also includes any visible representation made by means of any hoarding, wall painting, signal, light, sound, smoke or gas".

Amendment of section 23

In section 23 of the principal Act, for subsections (*2*) and (*3*), the following subsections shall be substituted, namely:

"(*2*) The name of the registered medical practitioner shall be reported by the Appropriate Authority to the State Medical Council concerned for taking necessary action including suspension of the registration if the charges are framed by the court and till the case is disposed of and on conviction for removal of his name from the register of the Council for a period of five years for the first offence and permanently for the subsequent offence.

(*3*) Any person who seeks the aid of any Genetic Counseling Center, Genetic Laboratory, Genetic Clinic or ultrasound clinic or imaging clinic or of a medical geneticist, gynaecologist, sonologist or imaging specialist or registered medical practitioner or any other person for sex selection or for conducting prenatal diagnostic techniques on any pregnant women for the purposes other than those specified in subsection (2) of section 4, he shall, be punishable with imprisonment for a term which may extend to three years and with fine which may extend to fifty thousand rupees for the first offence and for any subsequent offence with imprisonment which may extend to five years and with fine which may extend to one lakh rupees.

(*4*) For the removal of doubts, it is hereby provided, that the provisions of subsection (3) shall not apply to the woman who was compelled to undergo such diagnostic techniques or such selection".

Substitution of new section for section 24

For section 24 of the principal Act, the following section shall be substituted, namely:

"24 Presumption in the case of conduct of prenatal diagnostic techniques—Notwithstanding anything contained in the Indian Evidence Act, 1872 (1 of 1982), the court shall presume unless the contrary is proved that the pregnant woman was compelled by her husband or any other relative, as the case may be, to undergo prenatal diagnostic technique for the purposes other than those specified in subsection (*2*) of section 4 and such person shall be liable for abetment of offence under sub section (*3*) of section 23 and shall be punishable for the offence specified under that section".

Amendment of section 28

In section 28 of the principal Act, in subsection (*1*), in clause (*b*), for the words "thirty days", the words "fifteen days" shall be substituted.

Amendment of section 30

In section 30 of the principal Act, for sub section (*1*), the following subsection shall be substituted, namely:

"(1) If the Appropriate Authority has reason to believe that an offence under this Act has been or is being committed at any Genetic Counseling Center, Genetic Laboratory, Genetic Clinic or any other place, such Authority or any officer authorized in this behalf may, subject to such rules as may be prescribed, enter and search at all reasonable times with such assistance, if any, as such Authority or officer considers necessary, such Genetic Counseling Center, Genetic Laboratory, Genetic Clinic or any other place and examine any record, register, document, book, pamphlet, advertisement or any other material object found therein and seize and seal the same if such Authority or officer has reason to believe that it may furnish evidence of the commission of an offence punishable under this Act".

Insertion of new section 31A

After section 31 of the principal Act, the following section shall be inserted, namely:

"31A. Removal of difficulties

1. If any difficulty arises in giving effect to the provisions of the Prenatal Diagnostic Techniques (Regulation and Prevention of Misuse) Amendment Act, 2002, the Central Government may, by order published in the Official Gazette, make such provisions not inconsistent with the provisions of the said Act as appear to be necessary or expedient for removing the difficulty:

   Provided that no order shall be made under this section after the expiry of a period of three years from the date of commencement of the Prenatal Diagnostic Techniques

(Regulation and Prevention of Misuse) Amendment Act, 2002.

2. Every order made under this section shall be laid, as soon as may be after it is made, before each House of Parliament".

Amendment of section 32

In section 32 of principal Act, in sub section (2),

i. for clause (*i*), the following clauses shall be substituted, namely:
"(*i*) the minimum qualifications for persons employed at a registered Genetic Counseling Center, Genetic Laboratory or Genetic Clinic under clause (2) of section 3;
(*ia*) the manner in which the person conducting ultrasonography on a pregnant woman shall keep record thereof in the Clinic under the proviso to subsection (3) of section 4";
ii. after clause (*iv*), the following clauses shall be inserted, namely:
"(*iva*) code of conduct to be observed by persons working at Genetic Counseling Centers, Genetic Laboratories and Genetic Clinics to be laid down by the Central Supervisory Board under clause (iv) of section 16;
(*ivb*) the manner in which reports shall be furnished by the State and Union territory Supervisory Boards to the Board and the Central Government in respect of various activities undertaken in the State under the Act under clause (*iv*) of sub section (*1*) of section 16A;
(*ivc*) empowering the Appropriate Authority in any other matter under clause (*d*) of section 17A".

chapter 11

The Prenatal Diagnostic Techniques (Regulation and Prevention of Misuse) Amendment Act, 2003

(14th February, 2003)

GSR 109(E)—In exercise of the powers conferred by section 32 of the Prenatal Diagnostic Techniques (Regulation and Prevention of Misuse) Act, 1994 (57 of 1994), the Central Government hereby makes the following amendments to the Prenatal Diagnostic Techniques (Regulation and Prevention of Misuse) Rules, 1996.

1. 1. These may be called the Prenatal Diagnostic Techniques (Regulation and Prevention of Misuse) Amendment Rules, 2003.
   2. They shall come into force on the date of their publication in the official gazette.
2. In the Prenatal Diagnostic Techniques (Regulation and Prevention of Misuse) Rules, 1996 (hereinafter referred to as the said rules) in rule 1, for subrule (1) the following subrule shall be substituted, namely:
   "(1) These rules may be called the Preconception and Prenatal Diagnostic Techniques (Prohibition of Sex Selection) Rules, 1996."
3. In the said rules, in rule 2, clause (d) shall be omitted.
4. In the said rules, for rule 3 the following rule shall be substituted, namely:

"3. The qualifications of the employees, the requirement of equipment, etc. for a Genetic Counseling Center, Genetic Laboratory, Genetic Clinic, Ultrasound Clinic and Imaging Center shall be as under:

1. Any person being or employing
   i. A gynecologist or a pediatrician having six months experience or four weeks training in genetic counseling or
   ii. A medical geneticists, having adequate space and educational charts/models/equipment for carrying out genetic counseling may set up a genetic counseling center and get it registered as a genetic counseling center.
2. a. Any person having adequate space and being or employing:
      i. A medical geneticist and
      ii. A laboratory technician, having a BSc degree in biological sciences or a degree or diploma in medical laboratory course with at least one year experience in conducting appropriate prenatal diagnostic techniques, tests or procedures may set up a genetic laboratory.
   b. Such laboratory should have or acquire such of the following equipment as may be necessary for carrying out chromosomal studies, bio-chemical studies and molecular studies:
      i. Chromosomal studies:
         1. Laminar flow hood with ultraviolet and fluorescent light or other suitable culture hood.
         2. Photomicroscope with fluorescent source of light.
         3. Inverted microscope.
         4. Incubator and oven.

5. Carbon dioxide incubator or closed system with 5% CO_2 atmosphere.
6. Autoclave.
7. Refrigerator.
8. Water bath.
9. Centrifuge.
10. Vortex mixer.
11. Magnetic stirrer.
12. pH meter.
13. A sensitive balance (preferably electronic) with sensitivity of 0.1 milligram.
14. Double distillation apparatus (glass).
15. Such other equipment as may be necessary.

ii. **Biochemical studies:** (Requirements according to tests to be carried out):
1. Laminar flow hood with ultraviolet and fluorescent light or other suitable culture hood.
2. Inverted microscope.
3. Incubator and oven.
4. Carbon dioxide incubator or closed system with 5% CO_2 atmosphere.
5. Autoclave.
6. Refrigerator.
7. Water bath.
8. Centrifuge.
9. Electrophoresis apparatus and power supply.
10. Chromatography chamber.
11. Spectrophotometer and Elisa reader or Radioimmunoassay system (with gamma-beta counter) or fluorometer for various biochemical tests.

12. Vortex mixer.
13. Magnetic stirrer.
14. pH meter.
15. A sensitive balance (preferably electronic) with sensitivity of 0.1 milligram.
16. Double distillation apparatus (glass).
17. Liquid nitrogen tank.
18. Such other equipment as may be necessary.

iii. Molecular studies:

1. Inverted microscope.
2. Incubator.
3. Oven.
4. Autoclave.
5. Refrigerators (4° and –20°C).
6. Water bath.
7. Microcentrifuge.
8. Electrophoresis apparatus and power supply.
9. Vertex mixer.
10. Magnetic stirrer.
11. pH meter.
12. A sensitive balance (preferably electronic) with sensitivity of 0.1 milligram.
13. Double distillation apparatus (glass).
14. PCR machine.
15. Refrigerated centrifuge.
16. Ultraviolet Illuminator with photographic attachment or other documentation system.
17. Precision micropipettes.
18. Such other equipment as may be necessary.

3. 1. Any person having adequate space and being or employing
    a. Gynecologist having experience of performing at least 20 procedures in chorionic villi aspirations per vagina or per abdomen, chorionic villi biopsy, amniocentesis, cordocentesis fetoscopy fetal skin or organ biopsy or fetal blood sampling, etc. under supervision of an experienced gynecologist in these fields, or
    b. A sonologist, imaging specialist, radiologist or registered medical practitioner having Post-graduate degree or diploma or six months training or one year experience in sonography or image scanning, or
    c. A medical geneticist may set up a genetic clinic/ultrasound clinic/imaging center.
   2. The genetic clinic/ultrasound clinic/imaging center should have or acquire such of the following equipment, as may be necessary for carrying out the tests or procedures:
    a. Equipment and accessories necessary for carrying out clinical examination by an obstetrician or gynecologist.
    b. An ultrasonography machine including mobile ultrasound machine, imaging machine or any other equipment capable of conducting fetal ultrasonography.
    c. Appropriate catheters and equipment for carrying out chorionic villi aspirations per vagina or per abdomen.
    d. Appropriate sterile needles for amniocentesis or cordocentesis.
    e. A suitable fetoscope with appropriate accessories for fetoscopy, fetal skin or organ biopsy or fetal blood sampling shall be optional.

  f. Equipment for dry and wet sterilization.
  g. Equipment for carrying out emergency procedures such as evacuation of uterus or resuscitation in case of need.
  h. Genetic Works Station.
4. In the said rules, for the words "Genetic Counseling Center, Genetic Laboratory and Genetic Clinic", the words "Genetic Counseling Center, Genetic Laboratory, Genetic Clinic, Ultrasound Clinic and Imaging Centers" shall be substituted wherever they occur.
5. In the said rules, for Form A, Form B, Form C, Form D, Form E, Form F, Form G, and Form H, the following forms shall be substituted respectively, namely.

FORM A

[See rules 4(1) and 8(1)]
(To be submitted in duplicate with supporting documents as enclosures)

Form of application for registration or renewal of registration of a genetic counseling center/genetic laboratory/ genetic clinic/ultrasound clinic/imaging center

1. Name of the applicant
(specify Sh/Smt/Kur/Dr).
2. Address of the applicant.
3. Capacity in which applying.
(specify owner/partner/managing director/other to be stated).
4. Type of facility to be registered
(Please specify whether the application is for registration of a Genetic Counseling Center/Genetic Laboratory/ Genetic Clinic/Ultrasound Clinic/Imaging Center or any combination of these).
5. Full name and address/addresses of Genetic Counseling Center/Genetic Laboratory/Genetic Clinic/Ultrasound Clinic/Imaging Center with Telephone/Fax number(s)/ Telegraphic /Telex/ E-mail address(s).
6. Type of ownership and organization (specify individual ownership/partnership/company/cooperative/any other). In case of type of organization is other than individual ownership, furnish copy of articles of association and names and addresses of other persons responsible for management, as enclosure.
7. Type of Institution (Govt. Hospital/Municipal Hospital/ Public Hospital/Private Hospital/Private Nursing Home/ Private Clinic/Private Laboratory/any other to be stated).

8. Specific prenatal diagnostic procedures/tests for which approval is sought:
   a. Invasive — Amniocentesis/Chorionic villi aspiration/Chromosomal/Biochemical/Molecular studies
   b. Non-invasive — Ultrasonography

   Leave blank if registration sought for Genetic Counseling Center only.
9. Space available for the Counseling Center/Clinic/Laboratory give total work area excluding lobbies, waiting rooms, stairs, etc. and enclose plan.
10. Equipment available with the make and model of each equipment (list to be attached on a separate sheet).
11. a. Facilities available in the Counseling Center.
    b. Whether facilities are or would be available in the Laboratory/Clinic for the following tests:
       i. Ultrasound
       ii. Amniocentesis
       iii. Chorionic villi aspiration
       iv. Fetoscopy
       v. Fetal biopsy
       vi. Cordocentesis.
    c. Whether facilities are available in the Laboratory, Clinic for the following:
       i. Chromosomal studies
       ii. Biochemical studies
       iii. Molecular studies
       iv. Pre-implantation genetic diagnosis.
12. Names, qualifications, experience and registration number of employees (may be furnished as an enclosure) (Refer Schedules I, II or III).
13. State whether the Genetic Counseling Center/Genetic Laboratory/Genetic Clinic/Ultrasound Clinic/Imaging

Center qualifies for registration in terms of minimum requirements laid down in Schedule I, II and III and if not, reasons therefore.

14. For renewal applications only:
    a. Registration No.
    b. Date of issue and date of expiry of existing certificate of registration.
15. List of enclosures:
    (Please attach a list of enclosures/supporting documents attached to this application).

Date: ——————— Name, designation and signature of the person authorized to sign on behalf of the organization to be registered

Place: ——————

DECLARATION

I, Sh/Smt/Kum/Dr...........................son/daughter/wife of .... aged..........years resident of .... working as (indicate designation) .... in (indicate name of the organization to be registered .... hereby declare that I have read and understood the Prenatal Diagnostic Techniques (Regulation and Prevention of Misuse) Act, 1994 (57 of 1994) and the Prenatal Diagnostic Techniques (Regulation and Prevention of Misuse) Rules, 1996.

I also undertake to explain the said Act and Rules to all employees of the Genetic Counseling Center/Genetic Laboratory/Genetic Clinic/Ultrasound Clinic/Imaging Center in respect of which registration is sought and to ensure that Act and Rules are fully complied with.

Date:—————— Name, designation and signature of the person authorized to sign on behalf of the organization to be registered

Place: ————

[Seal of the organization sought to be registered]

ACKNOWLEDGEMENT
[See Rules 4(2) and 8(1)]

The application in Form A in duplicate for grant*/renewal* of registration of Genetic Counseling Center*/Genetic Laboratory*/Genetic Clinic*/ Ultrasound Clinic*/Imaging Center* by .... (Name and address of applicant) has been received by the Appropriate Authority .... On (date).

*The list of enclosures attached to the application in Form A has been verified with the enclosures submitted and found to be correct.

OR

*On verification it is found that the following documents mentioned in the list of enclosures are not actually enclosed.

This acknowledgement does not confer any rights on the applicant for grant or renewal of registration.

(.......................................)

Signature and Designation of Appropriate Authority, or authorized person in the office of the Appropriate Authority.

Date:————

Place————

[SEAL]

* Strike out whichever is not applicable or not necessary.

All enclosures are to be authenticated by signature of the applicant

ORIGINAL/DUPLICATE FOR DISPLAY

FORM B

[See Rules 6(2), 6(5) and 8(2)]

CERTIFICATE OF REGISTRATION

(To be issued in duplicate)

1. In exercise of the powers conferred under Section 19 (1) of the Prenatal Diagnostic Techniques (Regulation and Prevention of Misuse) Act, 1994 (57 of 1994), the Appropriate Authority ………………….. hereby grants registration to the Genetic Counseling Center*/Genetic Laboratory*/Genetic Clinic*/ Ultrasound Clinic*/Imaging Center* named below for purposes of carrying out Genetic Counseling/Prenatal Diagnostic Procedures*/Prenatal Diagnostic Tests/ Ultrasonography as defined in the aforesaid Act for a period of five years ending on ……………

2. This registration is granted subject to the aforesaid Act and Rules framed thereunder and any contravention thereof shall result in suspension or cancellation of this Certificate of Registration before the expiry of the said period of five years apart from prosecution.

A. Name and address of the Genetic Counseling Center*/ Genetic Laboratory*/Genetic Clinic*/ Ultrasound Clinic*/ Imaging Center*.
B. Name of Applicant for registration.
C. Prenatal diagnostic procedures* approved for (Genetic Clinic).
   i. Ultrasound invasive
   ii. Amniocentesis
   iii. Chorionic villi biopsy
   iv. Fetoscopy
   v. Fetal skin or organ biopsy
   vi. Cordocentesis
   vii. Any other (specify)

D. Prenatal diagnostic tests* approved (for genetic laboratory)
   i. Chromosomal studies
   ii. Biochemical studies
   iii. Molecular studies
   iv. Any other (specify)

3. Model and make of equipment being used (any change is to be intimated to the Appropriate Authority under rule 13).
4. Registration number allotted.
5. Period of validity of earlier Certificate of Registration (For renewed Certificate Registration only)
   From .... To ....

Date:..................

Signature, name and designation
of the Appropriate Authority

[SEAL]

*Strike out whichever is not applicable or not necessary.

DISPLAY ONE COPY OF THIS CERTIFICATE AT A CONSPICUOUS PLACE AT THE PLACE OF BUSINESS

FORM C
[See Rules 6(3), 6(5) and 8(3)]

Form for Rejection of Application for Grant/Renewal of Registration

In exercise of the powers conferred under Section 19 (2) of the Prenatal Diagnostic Techniques (Regulation and Prevention of Misuse) Act, 1994, (57 of 1994) the Appropriate Authority .... hereby rejects the application for grant*/renewal* of registration of the Genetic Counseling Center*/Genetic Laboratory*/Genetic Clinic*/ Ultrasound Clinic*/Imaging Center*.

1. Name and address of the Genetic Counseling Center*/ Genetic Laboratory*/Genetic Clinic*/Ultrasound*/Imaging Center*.
2. Reasons for rejection of application for grant /renewal of registration.

Date: ____________ Signature, name and designation
Place: ____________ of the Appropriate Authority with

[**SEAL**]

*Strike out whichever is not applicable or necessary.

FORM D
[See rule 9(2)]

Form for Maintenance of Records by the Genetic Counseling Center

1. Name and address of Genetic Counseling Center.
2. Registration No.
3. Patient's name.
4. Age.
5. Husband's/Father's name.
6. Full address with Tel. No, if any.
7. Referred by (Full name and address of Doctor(s) with registration No.(s) Referred note to be preserved carefully with case papers).
8. Last menstrual period/weeks of pregnancy.
9. History of genetic/medical disease in the family (specify) Basis of diagnosis:
    a. Clinical
    b. Biochemical
    c. Cytogenetic
    d. Other (e.g. radiological, ultrasonography)
10. Indication for prenatal diagnosis
    A. Previous child/children with:
        i. Chromosomal disorders
        ii. Metabolic disorders
        iii. Congenital anomaly
        iv. Mental retardation
        v. Hemoglobinopathy
        vi. Sex linked disorders
        vii. Single gene disorder
        viii. Any other (specify)
    B. Advanced maternal age (35 years or above)
    C. Mother/father/sibling having genetic disease (specify)
    D. Others (specify)

11. Procedure advised*
    i. Ultrasound
    ii. Amniocentesis
    iii. Chorionic villi biopsy
    iv. Fetoscopy
    v. Fetal skin or organ biopsy
    vi. Cordocentesis
    vii. Any other (specify).
12. Laboratory tests to be carried out:
    i. Chromosomal studies
    ii. Biochemical studies
    iii. Molecular studies
    iv. Preimplantation genetic diagnosis.
13. Result of prenatal diagnosis Normal/Abnormal
    If abnormal give details.
14. Was MTP advised?
15. Name and address of Genetic Clinic to which patient referred.
16. Dates of commencement and completion of genetic counseling.

Name, Signature and Registration No. of
the Medical Geneticist/Gynecologist/
Pediatrician administering Genetic Counseling]

Date:____________
Place:____________

* Strike out whichever is not applicable or necessary.

FORM E
[See Rule 9(3)]

Form for Maintenance of Records by the Genetic Laboratory

1. Name and address of Genetic Laboratory.
2. Registration No.
3. Patient's name.
4. Age.
5. Husband's/Father's name.
6. Full address with Tel. No. if any.
7. Referred by/sample sent by (full name and address of Genetic Clinic) (Referral note to be preserved carefully with case papers).
8. Type of sample: Maternal blood/Chorionic villus sample/ Amniotic fluid/Fetal blood or other fetal tissue (specify).
9. Specify indication for prenatal diagnosis
   A. Previous child/children with:
      i. Chromosomal disorders
      ii. Metabolic disorders
      iii. Malformation(s)
      iv. Mental retardation
      v. Hereditary hemolytic anemia
      vi. Sex-linked disorder
      vii. Single gene disorder
      viii. Any other (specify)
   B. Advanced maternal age (35 years or above)
   C. Mother/father/sibling have genetic disease (specify)
   D. Other (specify)
10. Laboratory tests carried out (give details):
    i. Chromosomal studies
    ii. Biochemical studies
    iii. Molecular studies
    iv. Preimplantation genetic diagnosis

11. Result of prenatal diagnosis Normal/Abnormal
    If abnormal give details.
12. Date(s) on which tests carried out.
    The results of the Prenatal diagnostic tests were conveyed to .... on ....

Name, Signature and Registration No. of the
Medical Geneticist/Director of the Institute

Date: ____________

Place: ____________

* Strike out whichever is not applicable or necessary.

FORM F
[See Rule Section 4(3), rule 9(4) and rule 10(1A)]

Form for Maintenance of Records in Respect of Pregnant Women by Genetic Clinic/Ultrasound Clinic/ Imaging Center

1. Name and address of Genetic Clinic/ Ultrasound Clinic/ Imaging Center.
2. Registration No.
3. Patient's name and her age.
4. Number of children with sex of each child.
5. Husband's/Father's name.
6. Full address with Tel. No. if any.
7. Referred by (full name and address of Doctor(s)/Genetic Counseling Center Referral note to be preserved carefully with case papers/self referral).
8. Last menstrual period/weeks of pregnancy.
9. History of genetic/medical disease in the family (specify) Basis of diagnosis:
   a. Clinical
   b. Biochemical
   c. Cytogenetic
   d. Other (e.g. radiological, ultrasonography, etc. specify).
10. Indication for prenatal diagnosis
    A. Previous child/children with:
       i. Chromosomal disorders
       ii. Metabolic disorders
       iii. Congenital anomaly
       iv. Mental retardation
       v. Hemoglobinopathy
       vi. Sex linked disorders
       vii. Single gene disorder

viii. Any other (specify)

B. Advanced maternal age (35 years or above).

C. Mother/father/sibling has genetic disease (specify).

D. Other (specify).

11. Procedures carried out (with name and registration No. of Gynecologist/Radiologist/Registered Medical Practitioner) who performed it.

Non-invasive:

Ultrasound (specify purpose for which ultrasound is to done during pregnancy)

[List of indications for ultrasonography of pregnant women are given in the note below].

Invasive:

i. Amniocentesis
ii. Chorionic Villi aspiration
iii. Fetal biopsy
iv. Cordocentesis
v. Any other (specify)

12. Any complication of procedure – please specify.
13. Laboratory tests recommended:
    i. Chromosomal studies
    ii. Biochemical studies
    iii. Molecular studies
    iv. Preimplantation genetic diagnosis.
14. Result of
    a. Prenatal diagnostic procedure (give details)
    b. Ultrasound Normal/Abnormal (specify abnormality detected, if any).
15. Date(s) on which procedures carried out.
16. Date on which consent obtained (In case of invasive).
17. The result of prenatal diagnostic procedure were conveyed to ....on ....

18. Was MTP advised/conducted?
19. Date on which MTP carried out.

Name, Signature and Registration number of the
Gynecologist/Radiologist/ Director of the Clinic

Date: ___________

Place: ___________

DECLARATION OF PREGNANT WOMAN

I, Ms............................(name of the pregnant woman), declare that by undergoing ultrasonography/image scanning, etc. I do not want to know the sex of my fetus.

Signature/Thumb impression of pregnant woman

DECLARATION OF DOCTOR/PERSON CONDUCTING ULTRASONOGRAPHY/IMAGE SCANNING

I, ...(name of the person conducting ultrasonography/image scanning), declare that while conducting ultrasonography/image scanning on Ms.....................(name of the pregnant woman), I have neither detected nor disclosed the sex of her fetus to any body in any manner.

Name and signature of the person conducting ultrasonography/image scanning/Director or owner of genetic clinic/ultrasound clinic/imaging center

Important notes

i. Ultrasound is not indicated/advised/performed to determine the sex of fetus except for diagnosis of sex-linked disease such as Duchenne Muscular Dystropy, Hemophilia A and B, etc.
ii. During, pregnancy Ultrasonography should only be performed when indicated. The following is the representative list of indications for ultrasound during pregnancy:
   1. To Diagnose intra uterine and/or ectopic pregnancy and confirm viability.
   2. Estimation of gestational age(dating).
   3. Detection of number of fetuses and their chorionicity.
   4. Suspected pregnancy with IUCD in situ or suspected pregnancy following contraceptive failure/MTP failure.
   5. Vaginal bleeding/leaking.
   6. Follow-up of cases of abortion.

7. Assessment of cervical canal and diameter of internal os.
8. Discrepancy between uterine size and period of amenorrhea.
9. Any suspected adenexal or uterine pathology/ abnormality.
10. Detection of chromosomal abnormalities, fetal structural defects and other abnormalities and their follow-up.
11. To evaluate fetal presentation and position.
12. Assessment of liquor amnii.
13. Preterm labour/preterm premature rupture of membranes.
14. Evaluation of placental position, thickness, grading and abnormalities (placenta praevia, retroplacental hemorrhage, abnormal adherence, etc.)
15. Evaluation of umbilical cord presentation, insertion, nuchal encirclement, number of vessels and presence of true knot.
16. Evaluation of previous Cesarean Section scars.
17. Evaluation of fetal growth parameters, fetal weight and fetal well being.
18. Color flow mapping and duplex Doppler studies.
19. Ultrasound guided procedures such as medical termination of pregnancy, external cephalic version, etc. and their flow-up.
20. Adjunct to diagnostic and therapeutic invasive interventions such as chorionic villus sampling (CVS), ammnicentesis, fetal blood smapling, fetal skin biopsy, amnioinfusion, intrauterine infusion, placement of shunts, etc.
21. Observation of intra partum events.

22. Medical/surgical conditions complicating pregnancy.
23. Research/scientific studies in recognized institutions.

Person conducting ultrasonography on a pregnant woman shall keep complete record thereof in the clinic/center in Form F and any deficiency or inaccuracy found therein shall amount to contravention of provisions of section 5 or section 6 of the Act, unless contrary is proved by the persons conducting such ultrasonography.

FORM G
[See Rule 10]

FORM OF CONSENT
(For invasive techniques)

I, ... wife/daughter of .... Age .... years residing at .... hereby state that I have been explained fully the probable side effects and after effects of the prenatal diagnostic procedures.

I wish to undergo the preimplantation/prenatal diagnostic technique/test /procedures in my own interest to find out the possibility of any abnormality (i.e. disease/deformity or disorder) in the child I am carrying.

I undertake not to terminate the pregnancy if the prenatal procedure/technique/test conducted show the absence of disease/deformity or disorders.

I understand that the sex of the fetus will not be disclosed to me.

I understand that breach of this undertaking will make me liable to penalty as prescribed in the Prenatal Diagnostic Techniques (Regulation and Prevention of Misuse) Act, 1994 (57 of 1994) and rule framed thereunder.

Date: ____________ Signature of pregnant women

Place: ____________

I have explained the contents of the above to the patient and her companion……….. (Name ……………………………..
Address …………………………… Relationship …………..)
in a language she/they understand.

Name, Signature and Registration number of
gynecologist/ Medical geneticist/ Radiologist/
Pediatrician/Director of the Clinic/Center/Laboratory

Date: ____________

Name, Address and Registration number of
Genetic Clinic/Institute

[SEAL]

FORM H

[See Rule 9(5)]

Form for Maintenance of Permanent Record of Applications for Grant/Rejection of Registration Under the Prenatal Diagostic Techniques (Regulation and Prevention of Misuse) Act, 1994

1. Sl. No.
2. File number of Appropriate Authority.
3. Date of receipt of application for grant of registration.
4. Name, Address, Phone/Fax, etc. of Applicant.
5. Name and address(es) of Genetic Counseling Center*/ Genetic Laboratory*/Genetic Clinic*/Ultrasound Clinic*/ Imaging Center*.
6. Date of consideration by Advisory Committee and recommendation of Advisory Committee, in summary.
7. Outcome of application (state granted/rejected and date of issue of orders record date of issue of order in Form B or Form C).
8. Registration number allotted and date of expiry of registration.
9. Renewals (date of renewal and renewed up to).
10. File number in which renewals dealt.
11. Additional information, if any.

Name, Designation and Signature of
Appropriate Authority

Guidance for appropriate authority

a. Form H is a permanent record to be maintained as a register, in the custody of the Appropriate Authority.
b. *Means strike out whichever is not applicable.
c. Against item 7, record date of issue of order in Form B or Form C.
d. On renewal, the Registration Number of the Genetic Counseling Center/Genetic Laboratory/Genetic Clinic/ Ultrasound Clinic/ Imaging Center will not change. A fresh registration Number will be allotted in the event of change of ownership or management.
e. Registration number shall not be allotted twice.
f. Each Genetic Counseling Center/Genetic Laboratory/ Genetic Clinic/ Ultrasound Clinic/ Imaging Center may be allotted a folio consisting of two pages of the Register for recording Form H.
g. The space provided for 'additional information' may be used for recording suspension, cancellations, rejection of application for renewal, change of ownership/management, outcome of any legal proceedings, etc.
h. Every folio (i.e. 2 pages) of the Register shall be authenticated by signature of the Appropriate Authority with date, and every subsequent entry shall also be similarly authenticated.

SCHEDULE I
[See Rule 3(1)]

Requirements for Registration of a Genetic Counseling Center

A. PLACE

A room with an area of seven (7) square meters.

B. EQUIPMENT

Educational charts/models.

C. EMPLOYEES

Any one of the following:

1. Medical Geneticist.
2. A gynecologist with 6 months' experience, in genetic counseling, or having completed 4 weeks' training in genetic counseling.
3. A pediatrician with 6 months' experience in genetic counseling, or having completed 4 weeks' training in genetic counseling.

SCHEDULE II
[See Rule 3(1)]

Requirements for Registration of a Genetic Laboratory

A. PLACE

A room with adequate space for carrying out tests.

B. EQUIPMENT

These are categorized separately for each of the under-mentioned studies.

Chromosomal studies

1. Laminar flow hood with ultraviolet and fluorescent light or other suitable culture hood.
2. Photomicroscope with fluorescent source of light.
3. Inverted microscope.
4. Incubator and oven.
5. Carbondioxide incubator or closed system with 5% CO_2 atmosphere.
6. Autoclave.
7. Refrigerator.
8. Water bath.
9. Centrifuge.
10. Vortex mixer.
11. Magnetic stirrer.
12. pH meter.
13. A sensitive balance (preferable electronic) with sensitivity of 0.1 milligram.
14. Double distillation apparatus (glass).

Biochemical studies

(requirements according to tests to be carried out)

1. Laminar flow hood with ultraviolet and fluorescent light or other suitable culture hood.
2. Inverted microscope.
3. Incubator and oven.
4. Carbondioxide incubator or closed system with 5% CO_2 atmosphere.
5. Autoclave.
6. Refrigerator.
7. Water bath.
8. Centrifuge.
9. Electrophoresis apparatus and power supply.
10. Chromatography chamber.
11. Spectrophotometer and Elisa reader or Radioimmuno-assay system (with gamma betacounter) or fluorometer for various biochemical test.
12. Vortex mixer.
13. Magnetic stirrer.
14. pH meter.
15. A sensitive balance (preferable electronic) with sensitivity of 0.1 milligram.
16. Double distillation apparatus (glass).
17. Liquid nitrogen tank.

Molecular studies

1. Inverted microscope.
2. Incubator.
3. Oven.
4. Autoclave.
5. Refrigerators (4 degree and minus 20 degree Centigrade).
6. Water bath.
7. Microcentrifuge.

8. Electrophoresis apparatus and power supply.
9. Vortex mixer.
10. Magnetic stirrer.
11. pH meter.
12. A sensitive balance (preferable electronic) with sensitivity of 0.1 milligram.
13. Double distillation apparatus (glass).
14. PCR machine.
15. Refrigerated centrifuge.
16. UV Illuminator with photographic attachment or other documentation system.
17. Precision micropipettes.
18. Such other equipment as may be necessary.

C. EMPLOYEES

1. A Medical Geneticist.
2. A laboratory technician having a BSc. degree in Biological Sciences or a degree or a diploma in medical laboratory course with at least one year's experience in conducting appropriate prenatal diagnostic tests.

SCHEDULE III
[See Rule 3(1)]

Requirements for Registration of a Genetic Clinic

A. PLACE

A room with an area of twenty (20) square metres with appropriate aseptic arrangements.

B. EQUIPMENT

1. Equipment and accessories necessary for carrying out clinical examination by an obstetrician/gynecologist.
2. Equipment, accessories necessary for other facilities required for operations envisaged in the Act.
   a. An ultrasonography machine*.
   b. Appropriate catheters and equipment for carrying out chorionic villi aspirations per vagina or per abdomen*.
   c. Appropriate sterile needles for amnicentesis or cordocentesis*.
   d. A suitable fetoscope with appropriate accessories for fetoscopy, fetal skin or organ biopsy or fetal blood sampling shall be optional.
   (*These constitute the minimum requirement of equipment for conducting the relevant procedure)
3. Equipment for dry and wet sterilization.
4. Equipment for carrying out emergency procedures such as evacuation of uterus or resuscitation in case of need.

C. EMPLOYEES

1. A gynecologist with adequate experience in prenatal diagnostic procedures (should have performed at least 20 procedures under supervision of a gynecologist

experienced in the procedure which is going to be carried out, for example chorionic villi biopsy, amniocentesis, cordocentesis and others indicated at B above).

2. A Radiologist or Registered Medical Practitioner for carrying out ultrasonography. The required experience shall be 100 cases under supervision of a similarly qualified person experienced in these techniques.

Note: In the said rules, Schedule I, Schedule II and Schedule III shall be omitted.

"Let us pledge today to remove gender bias from the scoiety and plea for uplifting of women"

At the end I would like to quote
Guru Nanak ji word's
"SO KEYON MANDA AKHYAE–
JITT JAME RAJAN"
means why the women be condemned
who have given birth to great saints, kings,
scientist and great leaders and **she is janani of all.**

Index

R

S

V

W